Nature's Virus Killers

NATURE'S VIRUS KILLERS

Mark Stengler, N.D., CHT, HHP
"The Natural Physician"

with Arden Moore

M. Evans and Company, Inc.
New York

M. Evans and Company, Inc.
216 East 49th Street
New York, New York 10017

Library of Congress Cataloging-in-Publication Data

Stengler, Mark.
    Nature's virus killers / by Mark Stengler.
        p.   cm.
    ISBN 0-87131-898-9
    1. Virus diseases—Alternative treatment. 2. Naturopathy. I. Title.
    RC114.5 .S74 2000
    616.9'2506—dc21   99-053637

Book design by Rik Lain Schell

Cartoons by Mel Schoneberger

Printed in Canada

9   8   7   6   5   4   3   2   1

CONTENTS

ACKNOWLEDGMENTS

A special thanks to my very patient and supportive wife, Angela. To our son, Mark Jr., who gave me lots of much needed breaks by running into my office while working on this book. To Dr. Jason Schneider, for his research assistance on the first two chapters of the book. To my talented editor Arden—thanks for the great work. Mel Schoenberger for his great cartoon drawings. To my patients, from whom I learn every day.

INTRODUCTION

~~~~~~

This book is about power. And control. And fighting back. You can gain all three through knowledge.

How many times have you found yourself sitting on that cold stainless steel table inside a doctor's exam room feeling miserable from a cold, the flu, or other health condition? After the exam, the doctor tells you, "It's a viral infection. There's really nothing I can do except tell you to get some rest, drink plenty of fluids, and wait it out."

You exit the office feeling powerless—and still miserable.

In *Nature's Virus Killers,* I'll teach you about all the formidable weapons you possess that can duel—and often, defeat—viral invaders. I'll guide you into a program to get your immune system in super shape, so that you can dodge the latest "bug" hitting your co-workers at the office.

Yes, the enemy is out there. Thousands of viruses are floating all around you every minute of every day. They are constantly searching for weak prey to penetrate. Some viruses wiggle inside bodies, but are soundly defeated by armies of immune cells. Other viruses victoriously overtake bodies whose armies are too busy fighting other fronts triggered by constant stress, poor diets, and lack of exercise. The most mighty and stubborn fleet of viruses can initiate cancer cells or develop into AIDS inside some victims.

A few viruses may actually deserve a welcome mat into the body—like chicken pox. You may be surprised to learn that antibiotics have no effect against viruses. Resaon for concern? Read on.

So, what are your allies in this war on viruses? Nature. Amazingly powerful and effective natural therapies stand ready

to assist you. Many of these therapies have been used successfully for centuries in European and Eastern cultures but are only
now being hailed as "the latest cure" by conventional doctors in
Western cultures like North America.

Every day, I witness these amazingly powerful and effective
therapies work their magic on my patients. A debilitating flu
can be knocked out within hours using natural remedies. Acute
ear infections can be cleared in minutes. A chronic viral infection like herpes that has nagged a person for years can disappear
within weeks of treatment.

The allies that answer your body's call to arms include
herbs, foods, homeopathy, acupuncture, hydrotherapy, vitamins, minerals, visualization, and mental imagery. They work
with your body's immune system to not only relieve the symptoms, but dig down and treat the underlying cause of the problem.

Let me illustrate. A common reason why some people are
prone to colds is because they eat too much refined sugar in
their diet. Large quantities of refined sugar are anything but a
sweet deal for your body. They rob your immune system of
needed nutrients, making it unable to fend off an invasion by
cold viruses.

Conventional medicine calls for taking over-the-counter
medications or prescriptions, but the cold virus doesn't budge.
The person sneezes, coughs, and wheezes for days.

The natural remedy game plan is much more complete. By
reducing the intake of refined sugar and adding more organic
foods and vital supplements to the diet, the person is better
equipped to stop the symptoms and the cold virus. The next
time the cold bug is going around, the body now has an impen-
etrable shield.

Natural therapies work at the cause and they do so with little to no harmful side effects. Think about that. How many times
have you read sentence upon sentence of cautions and warnings
on the label of a prescription bottle or over-the-counter medication packet? You feel like you're trading off one aspect of your
health for another. Why resolve one crisis at the price of harming various organs and structures in your body?

INTRODUCTION

In this book, you will discover how natural therapies can give you more of a role in your health care. Instead of feeling helpless, you can become a partner with your natural health-care practitioner to customize a battle plan that meets your specific health needs.

Most of the recommendations in this book are compatible with conventional therapies. They work with—not against—conditions that require prescriptions.

In summary, all therapies addressed in *Nature's Virus Killers* are designed to enhance—not weaken—your immune system. Not only do they help you in times of need, but they also help prevent you from being infected.

It all goes back to power. And control. And fighting back. This book arms you with the knowledge to take charge of your own health and harness the very power of nature for your own personal use.

Yours in good health and vitality,

Mark Stengler N.D., CHT, HHP
"The Natural Physician"

Chapter 1

VIRUSES: NATURAL BORN KILLERS

~~~~~~

What is a virus?
How does a virus invade a cell?
What's the difference between a virus and bacteria?
What are some common viruses?
Why are antibiotics powerless against viruses?
What are antiviral agents?

In their earliest forms, viruses were harmless messengers delivering hereditary information from newly developed life to its offspring in plants, fungi, protozoa, animals, and eventually people.

As viruses evolved and adapted to environmental changes around them, they ceded their messenger roles to cells and took on a more sinister role of infecting genes. In fact, virus is the Latin word for poison.

Some viral infections are short-lived: colds, the flu, sore throats. Others are lifelong: hepatitis and AIDS (caused by the human immunodeficiency virus). Collectively, viral infections represent the prime reason people visit doctors for medical care.

Throughout history, viral epidemics have plagued mankind and proven more powerful than the mightiest of armies. A flu epidemic wiped out Charlemagne's army in 876 A.D. Thousands of American colonists in the 1720s died after being exposed to a flu virus. The Spanish flu of 1918 killed more than 22 million people worldwide. The Hong Kong flu killed more than 70,000

NATURE'S VIRUS KILLERS

Americans in the late 1960s. In the early 1980s, a new viral disease surfaced that still plagues us today: AIDS. In the late 1990s, a lethal, fast-killing virus garnered headlines: Ebola. Like AIDS, there is still no cure for Ebola. Today hepatitis has become a major concern as well.

A virus is really little more than a clump of genetic material (DNA or RNA) bunched inside a protein packet. It needs a host cell to survive. Without one, it lies dormant. However, once it infiltrates a living cell within a person, it taps into that cell's reproductive equipment to duplicate itself. It makes thousands of copies of itself and, in the process, damages or destroys the host cells.

All this cellular debris and loose viral particles signals your immune system to fight back. White blood cells zoom to the infected scene, releasing chemical toxins, fever stimulators, and other agents built to fight invading viruses. Viruses test your body's infection-fighting capacity. As a consequence, symptoms including pain, redness, swelling, heat, fever, and rash often result. Because a virus is essentially composed only of genetic material, you can see how destroying it can be so challenging.

Fear not. Natural medicine features an arsenal of many solutions. Several years ago, Dr. Yuanhai He, a medical colleague of mine, expressed surprise while watching the television news. Airing was a story about a famous singer who had contracted hepatitis C. After attempts using conventional medicine didn't ease her symptoms, she said she was too weak to continue and was announcing her retirement from show business. She was frustrated because conventional medicine offered no solutions. This situation startled Dr. He. "That's so strange. Why didn't they try Chinese herbs and acupuncture to help her?" he asked. "In China, we routinely treat viral infections like hepatitis with these methods."

Why indeed. This book teaches you how to take a more active role in maintaining good health. The first step is achieved by understanding how a virus forms. I've provided cartoon illustrations in this chapter to help with the explanation. Subsequent diagrams will demonstrate how a virus duplicates, how it differs from bacteria, and how it can elude the immune system. The chapter concludes by providing you with insight into some of the more common and prevalent types of viruses affecting us today.

Viral Structure

The basic structure of a virus is quite simple. Viruses consist of a nucleic acid (DNA or RNA) enclosed within a protein coat (capsid) and they may or may not be enclosed by a cellular envelope.

Viral Replication in Host Cells

The virus, though simple in structure, entirely depends on our cells to supply the machinery necessary to produce more viruses.

How do viruses enter, replicate, and damage our cells?

1. *A virus has a special structure located on its outer surface that allows it to attach to our cells at special sites (receptors).*
2. *Once the virus attaches to the cell, the virus then enters the cell.*
3. *Within the cell, the virus sheds its capsid. Then nucleic acid is released into the cell.*
4. *The virus then uses the cell's components to replicate viral parts and to aid in the virus assembly.*
5. *After the new viruses are assembled, they can exit the host cell by one of three ways: by budding off the cell membrane (enveloped virus), cellular destruction (non-enveloped virus), or crossing junctions between cells.*
6. *The new viruses are now ready to infect other cells.* [3]

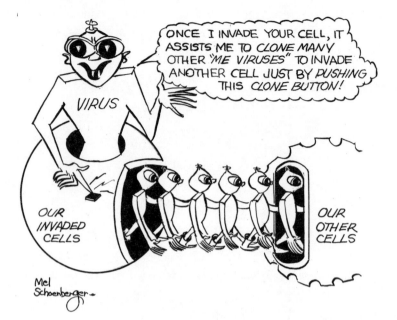

More dangerous than bacteria?

It is easy to confuse a virus with bacteria, but they are different types of foreign invaders. True, both have the power to cause an infection. Viral infections tend to be more widespread. Bacterial infections usually are more localized. A middle-ear infection is a common example of a bacterial infection. So is that redness and swelling you notice on a finger cut that was not properly cleaned.

In most cases, your immune system cells quickly fend off a bacterial invasion by simply surrounding and engulfing the bacteria (a process called phagocytosis). Then these cells release chemicals that kill and dissolve the bacteria. Victory is obvious when the site has completely healed.

The following table and diagrams help illustrate the distinctive differences between a virus and bacteria:

Bacteria vs. Viruses

Characteristics	Bacteria	Viruses
Size	0.5–1.0 micrometers in length and 10–20 micrometers in diameter	Smaller than bacteria. Some viruses can be living inside certain bacteria.
Mode(s) of Reproduction	• Binary fission (dividing into 2 new bacteria) • Budding • Branching	Parasitic (uses host cell to manufacture and assemble new virus).
Toxin Production	Yes	No
Intracellular/ Extracellular Infectivity	Both (outside and inside the cells)	Intracellular (requires cell machinery to make virus)
Cell Membrane Present	Yes	No

Bacterial Structure

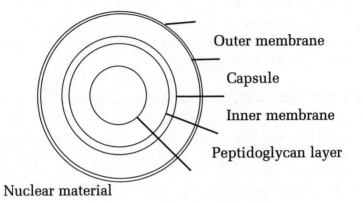

Outer membrane

Capsule

Inner membrane

Peptidoglycan layer

Nuclear material

Viral Structure

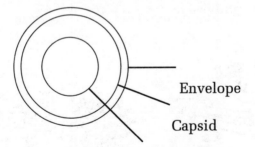

Envelope

Capsid

Nucleic acid

Mutation—the secret weapon of a virus

Viruses are stubborn and sneaky and possess a keen sense of survival. The following chart demonstrates how a virus attempts to bypass your body's built-in alarm system—the immune system.

Viral Evasion of Immune System Response

Viruses can avoid the immune system by several means:

Growing in areas where the immune system has limited access. Viruses grow or are shed into areas that are less accessible to the immune system (*i.e.,* cytomegalovirus [CVM] and the poliovirus in the digestive tract).

Surface antigen changes (mutations). Antigens are found on the cell membranes and tell the immune system which cells are infected. Viruses can alter their antigens, resulting in a delayed response by the immune system. This delay allows the virus time to replicate and assemble new viruses and increases its chances of further spreading the infection. Antigenic changes due to mutation result in a new infection from a different strain of the original viral infection. The new virus strain is relatively unsusceptible to the antibodies of the original viral strain. Mutation can also trigger latent or non-dangerous viruses to become lethal through alterations in the virus's nucleic acid. Persistence of a viral infection can be due to its ability to mutate into new strains and evade the immune system.

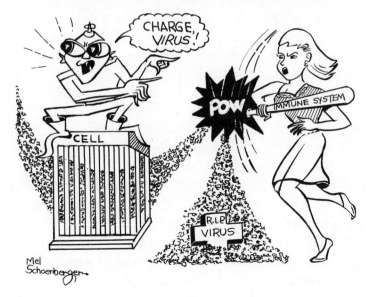

Suppression of the immune system. HIV and Epstein-Barr virus (EBV) infect the immune system, cause direct damage, and lead to the development of other infections (*i.e.,* HIV to AIDS).

About Certain Viruses

Viral infections range from the common cold to the nearly always fatal Ebola. This outline identifies some of the prevalent viruses we face today.

I. **Rhinovirus (common cold):** The rhinoviruses (over 100 strains) consist of a single-stranded RNA nucleic acid molecule and are not surrounded by an envelope. This virus is responsible for approximately 50 percent of common colds and only infects the upper respiratory tract. Once infected, our bodies make a specific antibody to avoid re-infection by this strain.

II. **Hepatitis viruses:** These viruses cause inflammation of the liver.
   A. Hepatitis A:
      1. *incubation period:* 30 (15–50) days [self-limiting infection]
      2. *severity:* mild to moderate
      3. *chronicity:* no
      4. *mode of spread:* fecal-oral contamination and close personal contact
      5. *carrier state:* none
      6. *chronic hepatitis development:* no
   B. Hepatitis B:
      1. *incubation period:* 90 (21–180) days
      2. *severity:* moderate to severe
      3. *chronicity:* yes
      4. *mode of spread:* blood (can live up to 2 weeks outside of body), blood products, sexual intercourse, close personal contact
      5. *carrier state:* yes (10 percent of infected)
      6. *chronic hepatitis development:* yes (5–10 percent of infected)

C. Hepatitis C:
1. *incubation period:* 20–90 days
2. *severity:* moderate to severe
3. *chronicity:* yes
4. *mode of spread:* blood, blood products, sexual intercourse, close personal contact
5. *carrier state:* yes
6. *chronic hepatitis development:* yes (greater than 50 percent of infected)

D. Hepatitis D:
1. *incubation period:* 30-50 days (requires Hepatitis B co-infection)
2. *severity:* moderate to severe
3. *chronicity:* yes (mainly due to Hepatitis B)
4. *mode of spread:* blood, blood products, sexual intercourse, close personal contact
5. *carrier state:* yes
6. *chronic hepatitis development:* yes

III. **Epstein-Barr virus (EBV):** EBV is responsible for infectious mononucleosis (IM). The virus has an affinity for the B-lymphocytes of the immune system. In IM, the infected individual has a fever, sore throat, enlarged lymph nodes throughout the body, enlargement of the spleen, and some liver impairment.

IV. **Ebola virus:** Ebola hemorrhagic fever was first discovered in Africa, in 1976. There are four types of Ebola virus that cause disease in humans. The Ebola Zaire strain is the most virulent, which is fatal in 90 percent of infected persons. Transmission of the virus is dependent on direct contact with bodily fluids of individuals or contaminated objects such as needles. The virus's incubation period is approximately 2 to 21 days; it will infect faster if there is a direct route to the bloodstream (*e.g.,* sexual contact). The primary response by the immune system is to produce anti-viral antibodies; unfortunately, they are relatively ineffective, and death results within 7 to 16 days. The specific cause of death is shock, often accompanied by severe blood loss.

NATURE'S VIRUS KILLERS

V. Hantavirus: Hantavirus was discovered in 1993 after outbreaks of an unidentifiable illness occurred in southwestern areas of the United States. It was found that people became seriously ill through rodents (mainly the deer mouse) that were infected by the hantavirus. The virus is excreted through rodent droppings, urine, and saliva. Thus, any contact with these contaminated substances can make one prone to infection. Direct contact with the virus can also occur through air that has been contaminated by the rodent droppings. The infected rodents have mainly been identified in rural areas.

The illness has an incubation period of 1 to 6 weeks. Symptoms of fever, headache, abdominal pain, muscle pain, nausea, vomiting, cough, and shortness of breath usually develop 1 to 5 days after the onset of symptoms. Respiratory failure and heart failure due to fluid buildup in the lungs can occur. A high fatality rate, of 49 percent nationwide, is reported.

VI. Influenza (Flu): There are three classifications of the influenza virus-A, B, and C. The most common cause of the flu is influenza A. It often occurs in epidemics during the late fall or early winter. The highest incidence of the flu is in schoolchildren. The incubation period is 48 hours. Acute symptoms usually subside in 2 to 3 days. Chills, fever, headache, and muscular aches and pains are the most common initial symptoms, followed by a severe cough. Persons at risk for serious complications include those with chronic pulmonary disease, valvular heart disease, or heart disease.

VII. Human Immunodeficiency Virus (HIV): HIV specifically attacks the immune system and allows other infections

and/or diseases to develop (*e.g.,* AIDS, fungal infections, pneumonia, etc.). HIV is known as an RNA retrovirus. It uses its RNA to make a double stranded DNA that then becomes part of the infected cell's DNA. Most viruses do not become part of the cell's DNA; instead, they use the cell's components/machinery to manufacture new viruses. The newly incorporated HIV DNA will then

22

be used to make new viruses, but it can be latent for months to years before the development of an HIV infection occurs. HIV depletes CD4+ T-helper cells, which are crucial in avoiding other opportunistic infections that will destroy other cells. Therefore, HIV sets the body up to be attacked by other infections, and with a very low CD4+ count, the development of AIDS results.

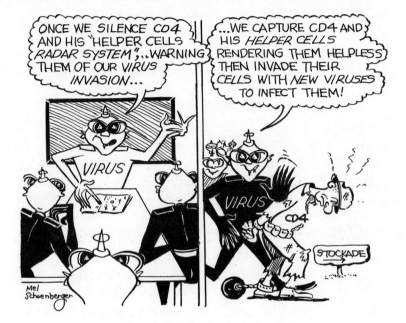

Effect of HIV on the Immune System

Treatment of HIV can be very difficult for two reasons:

HIV's RNA to DNA incorporation into the cell's DNA. The virus can be latent for months to years and then suddenly erupt.

HIV's immunosuppressive effect. HIV lowers immune system response and allows the expression of other infections and disease to arise. How can one increase immune system response when it is under attack?

Antiviral Therapy

What about antibiotics? Antibiotics cannot be used for viral infections since they work by destroying the cell walls of bacteria or by inhibiting protein synthesis within bacteria so they cannot multiply. Viruses do not have cell walls. (The envelopes and capsids are not cell walls).

There are many problems with the development of antiviral drugs:

- *Viruses live within the cells. It is difficult to get high levels of antiviral agent activity without damaging/destroying non-infected host cells.*
- *Timing. When symptoms of a viral infection appear, the viruses have gone through at least several cycles of replication. Therefore, the best time for antiviral therapy is at the initial stages of infection.*
- *Difficulty diagnosing viral infections. Viral infections can have vague symptoms, making it hard to decipher what type of infection is present.*
- *Many viral infections are relatively benign and self-limiting. It is important to weigh the effectiveness verses the toxicity of treatment in order to make the use of such agents acceptable.*

Current Antiviral Drug Therapies

DRUGS THAT BLOCK THE VIRUS FROM PENETRATING A CELL

One approach for drug antiviral therapy is to block the virus from penetrating the cell membrane. An example of a drug that is thought to have this action is amantadine. Although its exact mechanism is unknown, it is thought to prevent the virus from entering susceptible host cells. It has a specific use for the flu virus (influenza A). It must be given within 48 hours of the onset of symptoms to have any benefit.

VIRUSES: NATURAL BORN KILLERS

DRUGS THAT MIMIC THE IMMUNE SYSTEMS, ANTIVIRAL CHEMICALS

These types of drugs are designed to work in the same fashion as your immune system's antiviral agents to inhibit viral replication. To date, they are not anywhere near as effective as the chemicals naturally occurring in your immune system. Examples include:

Acyclovir—herpes, chicken pox, and shingles
Ganciclovir—herpes, cytomegalovirus
Ribavirin—respiratory syncytial virus
Vidarabine—herpes, chicken pox, and shingles

Another class of pharmaceutical antiviral medications are known as reverse transcriptase inhibitors. These are the drugs used for retroviruses like HIV. As explained on page 23, retroviruses like HIV are unlike most viruses in that they use the host-cell DNA (genetic material) to manufacture new viruses. Examples of drugs for retroviruses include zidovusine (Retrovir), didnanosine (Videx), zalcitibine (Hivid), lamivudine (Epivir), and stavidine (Zerit).

Your Body's Antiviral Artillery

The following are important components of your body's immune response to viruses:

Interferons (INFs) are found in the natural response by the immune system. They are messengers within the cell and have antitumor, antiviral, and immunomodulating effects. INFs' mechanism of action on viruses begins with binding to the cell membrane, in which it then stimulates the production of new cellular protein with an antiviral effect. INFs also inhibit cellular growth, enhance the cytotoxic effect of immune cells, and support antigen expression on the cell membrane.

Immunoglobulins (IMG) are the antibodies used to inactivate "free" viruses.

Future pharmaceutical antivirals

Researchers are trying to develop more specific agents that will affect viral replication mechanisms and are less toxic than present antiviral pharmaceuticals. One area of focus has been the viral DNA polymerase, which is required in order for the virus to replicate within the host cell. Studies of the effects of combinations of drugs are also being evaluated.[4]

Chapter 2

IMMUNE SYSTEM: THE BODY'S VIRUS KILLER

How does the immune system fight off viral invaders?
What makes up your body's first line of defense?
What makes up your body's second line of defense?
What role does fever play?

Every day, every hour, every minute, every second, the biggest battle of your life goes on right inside your body. Pathogenic disease-producers like viruses and bacteria are everywhere—in the air we breathe and the food and drink we consume. Fortunately, your body's complex immune system enlists an elite, elaborate army on constant alert for invading germs.

Within this microscopic army battalion are specialized immune cells equipped to identify, target, and fire upon invading viruses. White blood cells zoom to the infected scene, releasing chemical toxins, deadly enzymes, fever stimulators, and other natural weapons to kill unwanted foreign intruders. Special proteins, called antibodies, step in to replenish your immune system. Essentially, your immune system features two lines of defense:

FIRST LINE OF DEFENSE:
- *Skin and mucous membranes*
- *Sweat glands*
- *Hyaluronic acid/hyaluronidase system*
- *Saliva*
- *Mucus*

- *Stomach acid*
- *Gut flora*
- *Bio-electric field*

SECOND LINE OF DEFENSE:
- *Non-specific immune cells*
- *Macrophages*
- *Lymphocytes*
- *INterferon*
- *Complement*

First Line of Defense

In the first line of defense, your skin and mucous membranes form your body's biggest shield. Your skin is your biggest organ and acts as a buffer against viruses. Mucous membranes secrete mucus, which traps pathogens and other particles. Your body also harbors about two million sweat glands, which release moisture to help cool your body temperature. These sweat glands contain secretions that are antimicrobial.

The skin cells contain mucus-like connective tissues which produce a watery/gel-like material. They prevent viruses and other pathogens from moving freely between cells. This watery, gel-like material remains sticky because of the action of hyaluronic acid, which is also secreted by connective tissue. This acid prevents cell penetration by invading organisms. Some organisms release hyaluronidase, an enzyme that causes the gel-like material to become less viscous, much like when gelatin dissolves in water. This allows the invading organism to pass through more easily. Don't worry. As you will learn in Chapter 3, herbs like echinacea prevent the liquefying effect of hyaluronidase.

Saliva, produced by three sets of salivary glands located inside the mouth, contains antibodies that resist microbes and help clean the mouth, tongue, and teeth. Tears also contain immune factors that help wash pathogens away.

Moving downward, your stomach aids your immune system

by secreting acidic juices, which not only digest food but provide a natural barrier to viruses and other pathogens like bacteria and parasites.

Throughout the mucous membranes, and to an even larger extent in the colon, good bacteria called "flora" help to maintain immunity and fend off microbes.

Finally, all body cells communicate with one another through electrical impulses. The end result is a bio-electric field for the whole body. Experts feel this field acts as an overall shield for the body. As you will also learn, therapies such as acupuncture and homeopathy are believed to have a direct effect on the bio-electric field.

Second Line of Defense

The second line of defense, acting like a back up platoon, also serves vital roles for your body. This team includes non-specific immune cells. As their name implies, they are not designed for specific intruders. Rather, these cells attack when provoked or are summoned to attack when notified by other members of the body's defense squad. They also issue alerts to a specific defense system to gear up for action.

Let's begin the introduction of this team, starting with the white blood cells, which act like your body's infantry. They march around the bloodstream constantly searching for invading microbes. There are many different divisions of white blood cells. Neutrophils are white blood cells that destroy bacteria, tumor cells, and cellular debris. Eosinophils and basophils are mainly involved in destroying parasites and allergy reactions.

There is a special fleet of white blood cells called lymphocytes. Lymphocytes could be compared to the U.S. Navy. These very special white blood cells are produced by bone marrow and matured by the thymus gland. Lymphocytes swim primarily through the lymphatic system, although they also circulate in the bloodstream and are part of the high-tech radar of the immune system. The lymphatic system consists of lymph fluid that comes from the extra fluid between cells known as interstitial fluid. It flows through lymphatic vessels that run alongside

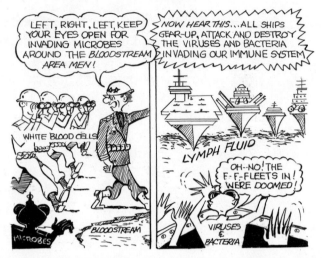

arteries and veins. Its movement is much different than blood flow. The arteries and veins move blood through the pumping action of the heart. The lymph is carried to lymph nodes, which filter the lymph through the action of macrophages. In addition, invaders such as viruses and bacteria are presented to B-lymphocytes in the lymph nodes for destruction (chow time, boys).

In addition, the spleen is an important player in the lymphatic system. This fist-sized organ is located behind the ribs in the upper left abdomen. The spleen manufactures white blood cells, destroys pathogens like bacteria, filters cellular debris, and destroys worn out red blood cells and platelets. It also secretes immune-enhancing compounds.

The tonsils and appendix are also localized components of the lymphatic system. Lymphocytes include T cells, B cells, and natural killer cells. A special type of lymphocyte known as the "B lymphocyte" produces antibodies, which bind to and "tag" a virus so that the rest of the immune cells can hone in on the invading microbe. The B lymphocytes are integral members of the specific immune defense team. As such, they react against specific intruders. Antibodies are produced in response to antigens, which are matter that the immune system recognizes as foreign, such as proteins found on a virus or bacterial wall. Antibodies are pre-programmed to react and attach to a specific substance, such as a type of virus. This signals the immune system to attack the intruder.

IMMUNE SYSTEM: THE BODY'S VIRUS KILLER

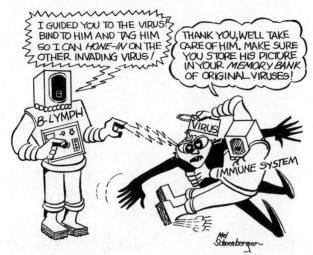

This is a very efficient system. Once the B lymphocytes encounter an intruder, they store information about this battle foe in their "memory banks" for future confrontations. Millions of antibodies then wait for the same intruder to return. Specific antibodies can also be massively produced—up to one billion a week—as needed to fight the same antigen recalled from the memory bank.

A specific type, the T4 cell, also known as the T-helper, is a fearless warrior savvy enough to seek and destroy viruses that hide undercover inside cells. It is involved in cell-mediated immunity, which means it does not react until another immune cell, such as a macrophage, presents a "target" to it. The T-helper

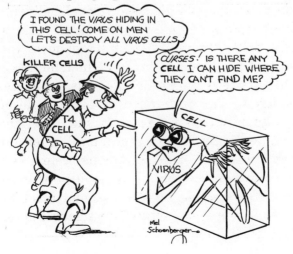

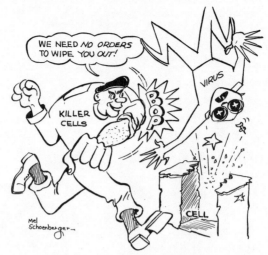

cells stimulate other cells such as macrophages and natural killer cells to destroy the target. Other T lymphocytes, such as T-suppressor cells, prevent the immune system from over-reacting, particularly against its own tissues. Natural killer cells, similar to a commando unit, attack and destroy cells infected with viruses as well as cancer cells. Natural killer cells also attack on their own and do not need directions from another immune cell to do so.

The last unit of white blood cells are the monocytes, which are the "janitorial" division. They clean up cellular debris after the immune system has battled an infection. They also play a role in triggering immune responses.

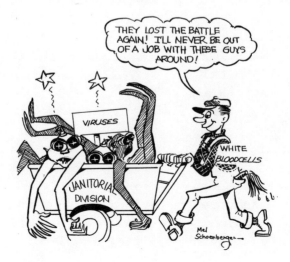

IMMUNE SYSTEM: THE BODY'S VIRUS KILLER

One type of white blood cell, called the macrophage cell, has earned the nickname, "the big eater." The macrophage hides in camouflage in tissues and organs and then eats invading microbes. Similar to a Pac-Man, it devours microbes, a process known as phagocytosis. It possesses a special weapon against viruses, known as interferon. Perhaps that name sounds familiar to you. That's because chemically synthesized interferon is often used in conventional medicine to treat cancer and hepatitis. But the natural interferon, made inside your body, is more effective. That's because your body's own interferon consists of a group of proteins that act like a team of special commandos. They are dispatched to specifically interrupt—and halt the spread—of viral growth. They also act like a radar system to alert divisions of the immune system to wipe out the invading virus.

If this wasn't enough, there is even more. When antigen-antibody reactions occur, a set of enzymes that circulate in the blood, known collectively as complement, is activated. This leads to a cascade of events that results in destruction of the intruding agent.

Summary of the key players of the immune system

This is by no means a complete summary of the immune system.

I. **White blood cells.** A group of immune cells that are designed to fight infection. These include:
   A. *Neutrophils,* which destroy viruses, bacteria, cancerous cells, and waste matter by surrounding and swallowing them. They comprise 60 to 70 percent of the white blood cells.
   B. *Eosinophils,* which are involved in allergic reactions and parasitic infections. In the later stages of infection and inflammation, they break down antigen-antibody complexes. They make up 1 to 4 percent of the white blood cells.
   C. *Basophils,* which are involved in allergic reactions. They comprise 0.5 to 1 percent of total white blood cells.

   D. *Lymphocytes.* There are several types of lymphocytes, which comprise 20 to 40 percent of the white blood cell count. These include:
   1. *T helper-cells*—help other immune cells to function.
   2. *T suppressors*—suppress excessive immune reaction.
   3. *Cytotoxic T cells*—attack and destroy viruses, cancer cells, and other foreign matter. They also secrete interferon.
   4. *B cells*—produce antibodies.
   E. *Monocytes* clean up cellular debris by removing dead cells, microorganisms, and other particles from circulation. They make up 2 to 6 percent of the white blood cell count.[1]

II. **Natural killer cells.** *Members of the body's second line of defense. They act on their own against foreign invaders.*

III. **Specialized cells and chemicals.**
   A. *Macrophages:* Monocytes that reside in the liver, spleen, and lymph nodes and destroy invading organisms and break down cellular debris.
   B. *Complement:* a collection of enzymes which enhance the immune response.
   C. *Interferons:* secreted by cytotoxic T cells, inhibits viral replication and draws the attention of immune cells to tumors.
   D. *Interleukins:* Many different types of this naturally produced chemical enhance the immune response.

Role of Fever in the Immune Response

Beyond your body's two lines of defense, is another hidden ally: fever. Many people automatically reach for an aspirin or acetaminophen to cool down a mild fever. As strange as it may sound, that may not be the wisest decision for your health. Studies have shown that aspirin and acetaminophen can suppress antibody production, decrease white blood cell production, and extend the length of cold symptoms.

IMMUNE SYSTEM: THE BODY'S VIRUS KILLER

You see, a fever is your body's inherent way of stimulating the immune system into action. When a macrophage devours an intruding microbe, for example, it releases a chemical, which stimulates the fever response. This, in turn, activates the armies of white blood cells and antibodies that fight off viruses as well as repair tissue and eliminate waste materials from your body.

A fever also initiates the withdrawal of iron from the blood (which microbes love to feed on) so that it can be stored in the liver and spleen. That's why it is important not to suppress a low-grade fever (registering 102 degrees Fahrenheit or below) by reaching for over-the-counter medications—it essentially prevents your body's immune system from doing its best job. This is best summarized in the textbook, *Human Physiology*, which states: "Fever is beneficial because it enhances the immune system's defenses, with all aspects of the engulfment and killing of invading organisms becoming more effective. Experiments with various warm-blooded and cold-blooded animals (the latter can increase body temperature only through behavioral adjustments) indicate that the ability to survive infections is greater if elevation of body temperature is not blocked. The conclusion: a fever is an unavoidable adaptive response. Many physicians now recommend that antipyretic drugs not be routinely prescribed to eliminate mild and moderate fevers."[2]

That said, any fevers registering above 104 degrees Fahrenheit (especially in children) or low-grade fevers that persist 3 days or longer should be considered dangerous and potentially life-threatening. You should seek immediate medical attention.

Note: Aspirin and salicylate medications (including the fever-reducing herb white willow bark) should be avoided in children and teenagers who have a viral infection, e.g., cold, flu. A rare disease known as Reye's syndrome can occur whereby a high fever, vomiting, liver damage, coma, and death can occur.

Immune System Response to Viral Infections

This antiviral battle within your body is complex. Allow me to walk you through the basics behind four key strategies.

NATURE'S VIRUS KILLERS

1. **Specific anti-viral antibodies** develop in response to viral infections and vaccinations. Specific antibodies interact with the viruses outside of the cells ("free") and make them inactive. They are prevented from entering the cells. Cells that are infected with a virus will display a marker on the cell surface (viral antigens). These marked cells can be recognized and destroyed by the antibodies, along with cytotoxic T-cells, natural killer cells, or macrophages.

2. **Cell-mediated immunity:** cytotoxic T cells and natural killer cells. Both of these recognize infected cells (by viral antigens on the cell surface) and destroy the cells before the viruses are assembled. This action prevents further replication and spread.

3. **Macrophage proliferation:** macrophages found at the site of infected cells discourage the formation of the bridges between cells. Macrophages can directly destroy the viruses by "eating" them along with infected cells.

4. **Viral-induced interferons** inhibit viral replication within the cells and prevent the spread to adjacent cells.[3]

The host immune system recognizes the presence of viruses and strives to destroy their breeding grounds (including host cells). This action ensures that non-infected host cells won't be infected and will be equipped to release interferon to block any further viral replication.

So, who wins the war—your immune system or the virus? Victory for the immune system depends on many factors. Your body has a tremendous innate ability to heal itself, especially when you keep it in optimal condition. Your choices and actions play pivotal roles. Eating a healthy diet (plenty of fresh fruits and vegetables and little or no refined sugars or fried foods); getting regular exercise (walking or doing some other form of aerobic workout for 30 minutes, three times per week); and limiting your exposure to environmental pollutants all serve to bolster your immune system. And don't forget about stress. Over time, your inability to handle stressful situations (from traffic jams to work deadlines) weakens your immune system.

In addition, the pathogenic strength of the intruding virus also plays a role in the outcome. As noted in Chapter 1, some types of viruses, such as HIV, have the ability to elude or even resist immune defenses.

Let's take the common cold as an example. The cold virus enters the body through the respiratory passageway. A macrophage eats the virus. This results in the release of interleukin (a chemical that signals the brain to raise the body's thermostat), and a fever results. Fever, as well as the secretion from the macrophages, stimulates the release of interferon (an antiviral chemical) as well as a host of white blood cells. T helper cells are attracted to the macrophages, which have sent out messages that an invader is present and pinpoint its location. The T helper cell also activates the B lymphocytes, which produce and attach antibodies to the virus. These antibodies attract other immune system cells to help out, like heat-seeking missiles. In addition, specific antibodies are established, so that the same viral strain will be recognized immediately in the future.

Chapter 3
HERBS: NATURE'S TOP VIRUS WEAPONS

~~~~~~

What herbs best fight viruses?
How do herbs boost the immune system?
How safe are herbs?
What's a virus cocktail?
What are the recommended dosages?

ortunately, Mother Nature provides an arsenal of medicinal herbs to assist your immune system in its fight against viruses. Echinacea, astragalus, reishi, lomatium, and licorice root head my list of the most powerful viral-fighting herbs. In addition, maitake (and other medicinal mushrooms), elderberry, olive leaf, and Saint-John's-wort exhibit strong antiviral actions. They also work wonderfully against flu viruses.

These herbs have proven track records for effectiveness and safety. They have been used all over the globe for centuries. The ancient Chinese and Greeks depended on these herbs to treat a host of viral-induced conditions such as colds, the flu, coughs, fevers, and hepatitis. The multi-medicinal benefits of these botanicals continue today. According to the World Health Organization, 80 percent of the world's population relies on herbs as a primary form of medicine. European medical doctors routinely use herbal therapies (known as phytomedicines).[1]

The best news: These popular herbs have successfully met stringent standards by leading scientists. In the past decade alone, there has been an explosion in the scientific validation of herbal medicines. Echinacea (also known as purple coneflower) is one of the most widely studied herbs. Tests have repeatedly demonstrated that one of its key ingredients, alkylamides, reduce inflammation and fever, and boosts white-cell production. White blood cells, as we mentioned at the beginning of this book, are part of your body's infantry, surrounding and eating foreign invaders such as bacteria and viruses. Another active ingredient in echinacea, polysaccharides, speeds production of a natural protein called interferon. This special protein is secreted by infected host cells to stop the viral invader from spreading to adjacent cells.

Astragalus, a mighty member of the bean family, has been shown to boost the immune system and inhibit certain viruses, such as the Coxsackie B virus. It has a long history of preventing and treating colds and various other respiratory-related conditions.

If you love mushrooms, reishi offers you an added medicinal bonus. The reddish-orange type is the best choice, because its polysaccharides contain the highest levels of immune-stimulating properties. It can be eaten as a food or taken as a supplement. Studies confirm reishi extract yields good results, especially in treating hepatitis and bronchitis.

Lomatium, a member of the parsley family, is a potent modulator of the immune system. It is a favorite amongst herbalists for treating colds, flus, and other viral infections.

Olive leaf extract has become a favorite to fend off a cold or flu. Different from the olive fruit, which prevents heart disease, olive leaf appears to have potent antiviral activity. I have had many patients report the beneficial effects of taking olive leaf extract for a cold or flu.

Genuine licorice root (not that red or black candy that shares the same name) has been a key ingredient in most Chinese herbal formulas for more than 3,000 years. Research indicates that licorice's two primary ingredients—glycyrrhizin and glycyrrhetinic acid—boost production of interferon. They also naturally inhibit the herpes simplex virus. The role of licorice root in treating HIV and AIDS is now being studied.

Primarily known as nature's answer to depression, Saint-John's-wort has been used since the days of ancient Greek physician Dioscorides for a variety of ailments. As for the history behind its name, there are many different legends. One version says that the red spots that appear on its leaves symbolize the blood of St. John, who was beheaded. Another tale is that if you tuck a piece of this plant under your pillow on St. John's Eve (June 24, the recorded birth of St. John the Baptist), the saint will appear to you in a dream, bless you, and prevent you or a loved one from dying in the following year. Regardless of its mythical roots, Saint-John's-wort has earned praise for its medicinal worth by scientists throughout the world. Two of its active ingredients, hypericin and pseudohypericin, are phytochemicals that display strong antiviral properties—enough to overpower herpes simplex viruses type 1 and 2, certain flu viruses (influenza A and B), and Epstein-Barr (the virus that causes mononucleosis).

When used properly, medicinal herbs offer specific advantages over pharmaceutical medications. They

- *cause few or no side effects,*
- *treat the cause of an illness, not just the symptoms*
- *prevent illness,*
- *can be used for more than one condition because of to their therapeutic effects.[2]*

The beauty of these herbs is that you can take them separately or together. They work in harmony with one another. In blending five specific herbs, I've created a "virus cocktail" formula that works on every viral condition from colds to herpes. These herbs supercharge your immune system. When combined with a healthy lifestyle and eating habits, and other natural therapies, these herbs deliver a more powerful viral-fighting punch.

Virus Cocktail

The "virus cocktail" is a potent herbal formula I developed in collaboration with Vlad Slama, a biochemist and noted herbal extraction research scientist from Kelowna, Canada. This cocktail attacks acute and chronic viral infections. It also provides an overall boost to your entire immune system. You can take it to prevent viral infections (especially after being exposed to someone with a cold). This formula—as well as similar formulas—

should be available in health food stores. Natural Factors is the brand that was used in our clinical studies and is available comercially. Or, you can grow or purchase these fresh herbs and combine them together to form a homemade "virus cocktail." Ingredients for my virus cocktail are:

- *Echinacea (echinamide)*
- *Astragalus*
- *Reishi*
- *Lomatium*
- *Licorice root*

To make a tincture (also known as a liquid extract) of these herbs, combine 30 drops of the first four herbs and 10 drops of licorice root to a half cup of warm water. Blend this combination. For acute infections, drink up to five viral cocktails daily. For chronic viral infections or for long-term immune system support, drink two cocktails daily. As mentioned, this formula should be available at local health food stores or pharmacies. A capsule form will work well also. A local herbalist or naturopathic doctor can also prepare this formula. (Note: To make a formula that works well against bacterial infections, just add 30 drops of Goldenseal to the virus cocktail.)

How well do these herbs work, separately or together? Let me share with you some success stories of my patients.

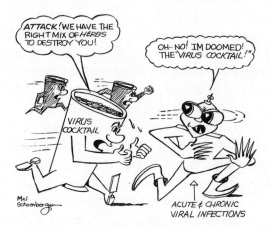

HERBS: NATURE'S TOP VIRUS WEAPONS

CASE HISTORY 1

Two years ago, Jane was diagnosed with chronic fatigue syndrome. Blood work indicated that she had a very active Epstein-Barr viral infection. Unfortunately, conventional medicine had little to offer, other than bed rest. Jane had to quit work. She spent most of her time at home resting and wondering if she would ever feel well again. That is, until one of Jane's friends, who happened to be a patient of mine, convinced her to come to my clinic and try a natural therapeutic approach.

Upon examination and after taking a thorough medical history, it was clear that, although chronic fatigue syndrome has many causes, Jane was definitely infected with the Epstein-Barr virus. Together, we worked on improving her nutritional status. I also prescribed to her my virus cocktail to help "kick" the Epstein-Barr out of her system. Within one week of being on the formula, Jane noticed that she had more energy and generally felt better. After one month of using the formula, she reported a 50-percent improvement. We kept Jane on the formula for four months, and she made a tremendous recovery.

CASE HISTORY 2

Many of my patients have benefited from the virus cocktail, especially Louis. This 70-year-old came to see me with a bad case of shingles. Shingles is a painful skin outbreak around the nerve pathways near the surface of the skin. It is caused by a reactivation of the dormant chicken pox (varicella) virus. It often occurs in the elderly when their immune systems are down. This condition can be quite debilitating. In addition to vitamin B12 shots, I put Louis on the virus cocktail. Within three days, his pain was dramatically better. Within two weeks, only slight remnants of the vesicles that had formed and blistered on the skin were present. This was a remarkable turnaround, considering that his shingles had been present for two months before he came to my clinic. The virus cocktail and, to some degree, the B12 injections strengthened his immune system enough to overpower the reactivated virus infection.

CASE HISTORY 3

Jim was a self-admitted type A real-estate agent. He had a high-stress job and was always on the go. He never took the time to eat properly, exercise, or get adequate rest. As a consequence, he was always getting sick with colds and respiratory infections. He came to me for advice on how to build up his immune system.

We talked about the importance of proper nutrition, exercise, and other lifestyle factors. Jim admitted that he didn't take the time to eat properly, exercise regularly, or practice stress-reducing relaxation techniques. He was also candid in stating that at this time in his life, he wasn't about to change his habits. He asked if he could take any type of supplement to reduce the frequency of his recurring viral infections. I introduced the benefits of echinacea to Jim and told him of the many scientific studies about it. I recommended that Jim take Echinacea daily for four weeks, stop for one week, and then repeat this cycle. This cycling technique prevents the immune system from becoming complacent from the immune-enhancing qualities of echinacea. Jim is still on the go, but he has fewer colds and respiratory infections now.

CASE HISTORY 4

Sarah, a 53-year-old teacher, developed a serious viral respiratory infection during chemotherapy treatments for her breast cancer. She came to my clinic for some natural help to boost her immune system. I told her that one dangerous side effect of chemotherapy is an increased risk of secondary infections because the immune system becomes so depleted.

The main herb I provided Sarah with was astragalus, which supports white blood cell production and the production of immune cells by the bone marrow. Sarah did very well on astragalus. Her oncologist noted that she developed a higher resistance to infections and avoided them during successive chemotherapy treatments.

CASE HISTORY 5

Linda, a 44-year-old receptionist, was diagnosed with HIV a few years ago. She came to me for dietary and herbal support after becoming very susceptible to upper respiratory infections. She would often need IV antibiotics to tackle these infections, many of which were a combination of viral and bacterial "bugs." As a safer, more natural alternative, I recommended that Linda take reishi extract. This herb from the Orient is known for its immune-building qualities. It is especially good for people prone to chronic infections.

Medical experts are divided over whether people with HIV and AIDS should take immunity-enhancing herbs. Some experts believe these herbs may actually stimulate quicker reproduction of the HIV virus (as the virus dwells within the immune system), but to this date, there has been no conclusive scientific study published showing this. Working closely with Linda's doctor, I had her take reishi extract daily for three weeks and then take one week off before resuming this cycle. Her doctor and I noticed that Linda's immune system improved and that she had fewer—and less severe—episodes of respiratory infections after taking reishi.

CASE HISTORY 6

When our son Mark Jr. was fourteen months old, he had a sore throat caused by a viral infection. I treated him with various homeopathic remedies and other natural medicines. On the second day of his illness, however, he developed a high fever that wasn't subsiding. This continued into the third night. My wife and I were starting to get worried because of the length of the prolonged fever. I finally gave him the virus cocktail. Within an hour of giving him two doses, his fever broke. By the next morning, he was back to normal and playing happily.

For the rest of this chapter, I will provide you with much more detail about each of these healing herbs. Summary charts are included to give you a quick reference. As for guidelines on how to take herbs and in which form, please refer to Appendix 2 in the back of this book. Special attention is given to echinacea because it ranks as one of the chief antiviral herbs.

NATURE'S VIRUS KILLERS

Echinacea

Pronounced *eck-in-AY-sha*, this herb has a long green stalk crowned with purple daisy-like petals and a cone-shaped seedy top. Echinacea is a hardy, easy-to-grow ornamental perennial that thrives in fertile, well-drained soil and prefers full sun to light shade. Prairies and open woodlands are its prime growing spots.

Plains Indians were believed to be the first to use echinacea, quickly discovering its medicinal benefits in easing colds and infectious diseases. Early American settlers learned to rely on echinacea as well, including it as an invaluable remedy for poisonous snakebites. By the 1870s, a Nebraska doctor popularized echinacea as a "blood purifier."

Nowadays, the words "colds" and "echinacea" are often spoken in the same sentence in many households. With the average American suffering two colds per year, it's easy to see how echinacea has quickly risen in recognition.

Actually, nine species of echinacea have been discovered. But a pair, *Echinacea angustifolia* and *Echinacea purpurea* are used primarily for medicinal purposes.

In Germany, physicians and pharmacists prescribed echinacea for the common cold for more than 2.5 million patients in 1994.[3] If herbs conducted popularity contests, echinacea would be crowned Herbal Queen. The fourth annual Whole Foods Natural Herbal Sales Survey ranks echinacea as the Number one selling herb, ahead of runner-up Saint-John's-wort.[4]

Researchers are still discovering how echinacea works. Evidence indicates that echinacea works in countless ways to support and boost the immune system, reduce inflammations and fevers, and increase white blood cell production. It also helps these cells to surround and destroy bacteria, viruses, fungi, and protozoa.

Noted herbalist and author Christopher Hobbs summarizes some physiological effects of echinacea in his book *Echinacea— The Immune Herb.*

Echinacea
- *Stimulates the leukocytes (white blood cells that help fight infection).*
- *Increases the "phagocytic power" of the immune cells (enhances the body's ability to dispose of bacteria, infected and damaged cells, and harmful chemicals).*
- *Inhibits hyaluronidase (which helps protect cells during infection, and prevents pathogens, bacteria, and viruses from entering in the first place).*
- *Provides a mild antibiotic effect.*
- *Stimulates the growth of healthy, new tissue.*
- *Delivers an antiphlogistic/anti-inflammatory effect (helps to reduce soreness, redness, and other symptoms of infection).*
- *Stimulates the properdin/complement system (helps the body control and prevent infections).*
- *Activates increased production of alpha-1 and alpha-2 gamma globulins (these prevent viral and other infections).*
- *Offers interferon-like action (helps prevent and control viral infections).*
- *Promotes general cellular immunity.*
- *Stimulates killer T cells.*
- *Inhibits tumor growth.*
- *Fights viruses.*
- *Fights candida (yeast infections).*[5]

About 400 scientific studies have scrutinized the chemistry, pharmacology, and clinical uses of this herb. Studies show that echinacea also slows the spread of infection to surrounding tissues and assists in flushing toxins out of the body. Several studies demonstrated concentrated compounds derived from echinacea activate macrophages, the germ-gobbling cells.

The majority of research has been done in Germany, where herbal therapy is part of mainstream medical practice. Many of the studies have been done in vitro (test tube) and on animals. Also, many of the published clinical trials have been done with an injectable form of echinacea. However, there is strong histor-

ical data on echinacea and some good studies using oral preparations of echinacea. Most of the oral preparation studies looked
at the prevention and treatment of colds and the flu.[6]

STUDY 1

Freshly pressed juice from *Echinacea purpurea* was studied to
see if it could prevent reoccurrence of colds in 108 people who
had a high susceptibility to colds. People selected had at least
three cold-related infections the previous winter. One group
received 4 ml (approximately 160 drops) of echinacea twice
daily, while the other group received a placebo. Blood tests to
measure immune function were taken at the beginning of the
study and at two other intervals. The groups were examined
after four weeks and eight weeks to see if a cold infection
occurred. Clinical results showed that people treated with echinacea had a decreased frequency of infections. They also developed milder infections and had a longer time interval before
their first infection (40 days), compared with 25 days for the
placebo group. Also, the echinacea group had fewer infections
spread to the lower respiratory tract.

After analyzing the data, researchers noticed that those people with weakened T cell (T-4) counts benefited from taking
echinacea. Those in the group who had a low T-4 to T-8 ratio (as
seen in HIV infection, one of the parameters to measure progression of this disease) had a dramatic reduction in the length
of infections from 7.5 to 5.3 days. Even though this is a small
sample size, it warrants further investigation into the use of
echinacea for those with HIV/AIDS.[7]

STUDY 2

A randomized, double-blind clinical study looked at the effectiveness of *Echinacea purpurea* tincture for people who had the begin-
nings of a cold. The 120 people in the study had experienced at
least three respiratory infections in the last six months. Half the
participants received echinacea. They took 20 drops in a half glass
of water every two hours for the first day and then repeated this
dose three times a day for 10 days. The other half received place-

bos. Patients recorded their symptoms and were interviewed by a physician during the course of their colds. Analysis showed that the group taking echinacea had a statistically significant quicker recovery time than people taking placebos.[8]

STUDY 3

This study looked at 180 people who were in the first few days of flu-like symptoms or feverish infection of the upper respiratory tract. One group received a placebo; the second took 90 drops (3 ml) of *Echinacea purpurea* root, and the third group received 180 drops of the *Echinacea purpurea* root. Symptoms of all participants were evaluated after three to four days and again after eight to ten days. The results showed that 90 drops of tincture was no more effective than the placebo, but 180 drops showed a noticeable effect, resulting in reduced length and severity of symptoms.[9]

STUDY 4

In a German study, test subjects took 30 drops of echinacea tincture three times daily for five days, while the control group took a placebo. The phagocyte (immune cells) activity was measured in the subjects' blood at the beginning and at certain intervals during the study. At day three, the phagocyte activity in the echinacea group had increased to 40 percent. By day four, activity climbed by more than 70 percent, and by day five, activity soared to 120 percent! When the dosage of echinacea was stopped, it took three days for the phagocyte measurements to drop and match the levels among participants in the placebo group.[10]

STUDY 5

Sports medicine specialists studied the effect of echinacea on male triathletes. It is known that triathletes are at an increased risk for infection due to exhaustive training. Participants took either a placebo, 43 mg of magnesium, or 8 ml of *Echinacea purpurea* for 28 days before the triathlon. During training, 3 of the 13 athletes in the magnesium group and 4 of 13 in the placebo group developed colds. Those taking echinacea developed no colds. Those in the magnesium group missed a total of 13 days of training while those in the placebo group missed a total of 24 days of training because of colds.[11]

STUDY 6

Not all studies of echinacea have been positive. An initial press release by Bastyr University on a 16-month, double-blind, place-bo-controlled study to evaluate the ability of *Echinacea purpurea* to reduce the frequency and severity of respiratory-tract infections stated there was no benefit to the supplementation to the group of users in the study. I cannot comment on this study since, to date, the data and specifics have not been released.

STUDY 7

A study suggested that common herbal supplements, such as Saint. John's-wort, ginkgo, and echinacea might adversely affect fertility. Researchers took hamster eggs, removed the outer coating, and exposed the eggs to the herbs. They then mixed in human sperm, which will usually penetrate the egg. At higher dosages, the herbs either impaired or prevented the sperm's ability to penetrate the eggs. High concentrations of *Echinacea purpurea* interfered with sperm enzymes.[12] Based on this, some researchers have prematurely concluded that echinacea may interfere with fertility. The media got a hold of this study and blew it out of proportion. Is this a valid conclusion? No; there are several problems with it. In the body, any herb is first broken down by the digestive system. In this study, the researchers used the whole herb in relatively high concentrations, which would never contact sperm in real life. Also, the experiment was done in a laboratory petri dish. To be valid human studies would have to be done, as there is often no correlation between what happens in a petri dish and what happens in the human body.

I could not stop laughing when I read this study and the portrayed conclusion, which was ridiculous. I have no problem recommending echinacea for short-term use in pregnancy or for those trying to conceive.

STUDY 8

A recent study conducted by the Hospital for Sick Children in Toronto, in conjunction with the Canadian Naturopathic College of Naturopathic Medicine looked at the safety of echinacea and pregnancy. A group of 206 women who used echinacea during pregnancy for upper respiratory tract infections were analyzed along with a control group of 198 pregnant women who had upper respiratory tract infections but never used echinacea. The researchers found no association with the use of echinacea and birth defects. There were also no differences in the rate of live births or spontaneous abortions between the two groups.[13]

Astragalus

This plant has been used medicinally as a prescription herb and food throughout China for thousands of years. It has become a favorite among western herbalists for its benefit to the immune system.

Although traditional Chinese medicine does not distinguish between viruses and bacteria, herbs are prescribed based on sets of patterns and symptoms. Using the Chinese medicine model, astragalus is used to strengthen the lung and spleen (the organ in Chinese medicine involved in digestion) meridians. It improves symptoms related to a spleen deficiency, such as lack of appetite, fatigue, and diarrhea. For lung deficiency syndromes, it is indicated for frequent colds and shortness of breath. Astragalus is said to strengthen the protective *qi,* which many western practitioners equate to the immune system. It is also effective against bacterial infections.

Many studies demonstrate the immune-enhancing effects of astragalus. Patients with viral myocarditis (viral infection of the heart) showed improvements in immune status when given astragalus extract. Astragalus is also used as an adjunctive herb in the treatment of cancer and to reduce the side effects of chemotherapy drugs.[14–19]

NATURE'S VIRUS KILLERS

Reishi

This antiviral herb is best known among the Chinese as *ling zhi* and among the Japanese as *ling chih*. Both cultures have used reishi mushrooms for more than 4,000 years to treat chronic hepatitis, enlarged liver, high blood pressure, arthritis, insomnia, neurasthenia, bronchitis, asthma, and gastric ulcers.

In the famous Chinese natural history book *Ben Cao Gang Mu* (1578), the authors wrote that "continued use of ling zhi will lighten weight and increase longevity." Professor Hiroshi Hikino, one of today's premier authorities on Oriental herbs, classifies reishi as one of the "most important elixirs in the Orient."

There are six different types of reishi mushrooms, all classified according to color. The red reishi mushroom is considered to deliver the most potent medicinal benefits. Asian studies report that reishi improves conditions among people with hepatitis and bronchitis. One study reported 60 to 90 percent improvement among 2,000 people with bronchitis, within two weeks of taking reishi.

Throughout its long history, there have never been any reports of toxicity or side effects from reishi.[20]

Lomatium

Herbalists regard this member of the parsley family as one of the most potent antiviral herbs. It is indigenous to the northwestern United States. Lomatium works very well for the flu, common cold, and respiratory tract infections. It is also an herb to consider using for urinary tract infections, herpes, and bacterial and fungal infections. One of the phytochemicals in lomatium, known as furnacoumarin, has been shown to block viral replication.

Olive Leaf

Ancient Egyptians used olive leaf extract to mummify their pharaohs. Nineteenth-century Britains relied on olive leaf extract to treat tropical diseases such as malaria. Today, scientists are still discovering the health benefits of this herb.

This herb is an excellent source of phytochemicals that provide powerful antiviral, antiparasitic, antifungal, and antibacterial properties. Researchers in the early 1900s were able to isolate a phenolic compound from olive leaves called oleuropein. Scientists determined that oleuropein was the ingredient that kept trees disease-free and resistant to insects. Olive leaf also contains flavonoids (including rutin flavonol, luteolin-7-glucoside flavone and hesperidin flavone) as well as elenolic acid.[21]

What does this mean? Well, these ingredients are mighty weapons against the common cold, the flu, and other respiratory infections. In addition, individuals who regularly take olive leaf extract report increased energy levels. Although there is not much in the way of human studies of olive leaf, I have had many people report tremendous benefit with its use in viral infections like the common cold and flu.

Olive leaf is available as a supplement in a capsule or tincture.

Licorice Root

The most common form of licorice root used in the western world is *Glycyrrhiza glabra*. In Chinese medicine, the most popular type is *Glycyrrhiza uralensis*. Licorice root has been used therapeutically for thousands of years. It possesses immune-stimulating effects as well as antiviral, anti-inflammatory, and anticancer properties.

One of its main active constituents, glycyrrhizin, is 100 times sweeter than sucrose. Two of the known active constituents, glycyrrhizin and glycyrrhetinic acid, activate interferon in the immune system, which has strong antiviral activity. Licorice root has also been shown to inhibit the growth of many viruses, including herpes simplex type. Topical applications work well in reducing the pain and healing time of both oral and genital herpes, and can be commercially as a cream.[22, 23]

Licorice root is commonly available in tincture, capsule, or tea.

Elderberry

This shrubby tree with musk-scented wood has enjoyed a reputation as a medicinal herb since the days of Hippocrates, the father of medicine. In seventeenth-century Europe, elderberry was dubbed the "country medicine chest" because of its ability to fight viruses and bacteria.

One legend tells of how the elderberry tree provided protection and warded off evil spirits. For centuries, people have picked its berries and made them into delicious wines, pies, and preserves.

Modern scientific studies report that key active ingredients extracted from elderberry provide the first line of defense against a viral invasion, especially by different flu strains. These ingredients neutralize new viruses released from invaded cells and prevent them from replicating themselves. Research performed in Israel showed that the juice from elderberries stimulates the immune system and inhibits the influenza virus. Patients with the flu have reported significant improvements within 24 to 48 hours, in contrast to those who received placebos and took six days to recovery.[24]

Not only is elderberry a great preventive against the flu, it also partners well with echinacea in dealing with colds and respiratory infections. Elderberry is available as a supplement in capsule or tincture form.

Larix

Larix is an extract from the western larch tree. It is used by herbalists and nutrition-oriented doctors for its immune-enhancing effects. One of the unique properties of larix is that it is very soluble. This makes it quite easy to use as a powder added to liquids such as water or fruit juice. Naturopathic doctors often use it with children for immune system support, as it has a slightly sweet taste and cannot be seen in liquids because of its high solubility.

One of the main active ingredients is a type of polysaccharide (long-branched sugar chain) known as arabinogalactan. Larix is often used for the prevention and treatment of colds, flus, and for ear infections.

Herbal Summary

- **Astragalus** (*Astragalus membranaceus*)
  Also known as *huang qi,* milk-vetch root.
  Description: Black roots with a pale yellow core.
  History: Used for centuries in traditional Chinese medicine as an immune tonic.
  Parts used: Roots
  Known active ingredients: Polysaccharides
  Actions: Boosts immune system.
  Medicinal benefits: Prevents and treats colds, and infections and provides support during chemotherapy and radiation treatments; treats bone marrow deficiency.
  Recommended dose: 20 to 30 drops of tincture or 500–1,000 mg capsule form three times daily.
  Cautions: Excessive amounts may cause indigestion.

- **Echinacea** (*Echinacea angustifolia* and *Echinacea purpurea*)
  Also known as purple coneflower, Kansas or Missouri snakeroot.
  Description: Purple cone-shaped native American wildflower, member of the daisy family.
  History: First used by Native Americans for a variety of medicinal uses.
  Parts used: Flowers, leaves, roots of *E. purpurea* and *E. angustifolia.*
  Known active ingredients: Alkylamides, polysaccharides, flavonoids, essential oils, polyacetylenes. There are nine species, with two used medicinally: *Echinacea angustifolia* and *Echinacea purpurea.*
  Actions: Boosts immune system, reduces inflammation and fevers, increases white blood cell production.
  Medicinal benefits: Colds, strep throat, staph infections, burns, herpes, skin ulcers, eczema, psoriasis, whooping cough, bronchitis, rheumatoid arthritis, allergies, toothaches, gum and mouth infections, bites, blood and food poisoning, boils, and abscesses.

55

Recommended dose: 10 to 60 drops of standardized extract tinctures or 500–1000 milligram capsules, three times a day.

Cautions: Generally safe. Avoid if allergic to marigolds or chamomile. Consult a physician trained in herbal medicine if you have an auto-immune condition such as leukosis, multiple sclerosis, lupus, or any collagen disease. Low potential for toxicity (but no reported cases in humans).

- ## Licorice (*Glycyrrhiza glabra*)

  Also known as sweet wood.

  Description: Long, cylindrical rootstock.

  History: Used for more than 3,000 years by the Chinese.

  Parts used: Roots

  Known active ingredients: Glycyrrhizin and glycyrrhetinic acid, flavonoids.

  Actions: Stimulates interferon production; inhibits herpes simplex virus.

  Medicinal benefits: Use for any viral infection or for digestive inflammation.

  Recommended dose: 20 drops or 500 mg three times daily, or as part of a formula.

  Cautions: High dosages (3,000 mg of powdered root or higher) may cause water retention, potassium loss, or high blood pressure.

- ## Reishi (*Ganoderma lucidum*)

  Also known as *ling zhi* and *ling chih*.

  Description: Reddish-orange mushroom with black body and slender stalk.

  History: First used more than 4,000 years ago in Japan and China to treat a variety of conditions, including chronic hepatitis, high blood pressure, and arthritis.

  Species: Six, classified by color, with the red possessing the most medicinal potency.

  Parts used: Fruiting body

  Known active ingredients: Polysaccharides

  Actions: Stimulate, immune system.

Medicinal benefits: Used for allergies, coronary heart disease, bronchitis, tumors, inflammation, viral infections, high blood pressure, HIV, and during chemotherapy and radiation treatments.

Recommended dose: 20 to 30 drops three times daily or eat as a food.

Cautions: Very safe; no side effects.

- ## Saint-John's-Wort (*Hypericum perforatum*)

  Description: Shrubby perennial plant with bright flowers.

  History: First used by Dioscorides and Hippocrates, famous ancient Greek doctors.

  Parts used: Flowering tops

  Known active ingredients: Hypericin, hyperoforin, pseudohypericin, flavones, xanthones, and essential oils.

  Actions: Powerful antiviral herb

  Medicinal benefits: Fights viral and other infections, cold sores, chronic fatigue, cough, depression and burns.

  Recommended dose: 300–900 mg of a standardized 0.3 percent hypericin extract, or 20 to 30 drops of tincture three times daily.

  Cautions: Photosensitivity (increase sensitivity to sun). Avoid use with antidepressant prescriptions.

- ## Lomatium (*Lomatium dissectum*)
  Also known as desert parsley.

  Description: Dissected leaves with white to purple flowers.

  History: Used by Native Americans and herbalists of the western United States.

  Parts used: Root

  Actions: Used for infections, particularly viral infections.

  Medicinal benefits: Antiviral against RNA and DNA viruses; used for Epstein-Barr virus, herpes, cytomegalovirus, and genital warts; Also good for respiratory infections and candida.

  Recommended dosage: 20 to 40 drops, two to three times daily.

  Cautions: In rare cases, users will develop a measles-like rash.

NATURE'S VIRUS KILLERS

- ## Osha (*Ligusticum porteri*)
  Description: Green stems with dissected leaves and white flowers.
  History: Treatment of respiratory infections by herbalists.
  Parts used: Root
  Actions: Antiviral; clears respiratory tract.
  Medicinal Benefits: Cold, flu, and respiratory infections.
  Recommended dosage: 30 drops, three times daily.
  Cautions: Do not use if pregnant.

- ## Shitake (*Lentinus edodes*)
  Description: Light amber fungi.
  History: Renowned in Japan and China as a medicinal food.
  Parts Used: Fruiting body
  Actions: Immune enhancement; antiviral (contains lentinan and Lentinula Edodes Mycelium—extract, which are strongly antiviral), antitumor, antibacterial and antiparasitic; protects the liver.
  Medicinal benefits: HIV/AIDS, hepatitis, cancer, candida, and bronchitis.
  Recommended dosage: As a food, 6 to 16 g of the whole dried fruiting body or as directed on container.
  Cautions: If using mushroom as a food it must be cooked, or digestive upset can occur. It is non-toxic, although rare cases of diarrhea and skin rashes have been reported.

- ## Maitake (*Grifola frondosa*)
  Also known as "dancing mushroom."
  Description: Fan-shaped caps.
  History: Highly regarded in Japan for its medicinal properties. Maitake collectors would keep their harvesting grounds a secret, as it was such a revered food.
  Parts used: Fruiting body
  Actions: Enhances immune activity: macrophage, natural killer cells, cytotoxic T cells, and has a special polysac-

charide called D fraction that stimulates interleukin1 (antiviral and antitumor effect).

Medicinal benefits: Immune deficiency conditions such as cancer prevention and HIV/AIDS, chronic infections, high-blood pressure, and diabetes.

Recommended dosage: Often eaten as a food. Take 3 to 7 grams a day, or take as a capsule as directed on container.

Cautions: None

- **Wild Indigo (*Baptisia tinctora*)**

  Description: Yellow brown root with fibrous stock.

  History: Used by herbalists for toxic infections, especially of the throat.

  Parts used: Roots and leaves

  Actions: Stimulates white blood cell destruction of viruses and bacteria.

  Medicinal benefits: Infected wounds, ulcers, lymphatic infections, tonsillitis, and sore throats.

  Recommended dosage: Use only under the guidance of an herbalist or a doctor knowledgeable in herbal medicine.

  Cautions: Do not use more than the recommended dosage, as larger dosages can be toxic.

- **Olive Leaf (*Olea Europaea*)**

  Description: Leaf of the olive tree.

  History: Used in the nineteenth century for the treatment of fever.

  Parts used: Leaf

  Known active constituents: Oleopurein

  Actions: Contains the chemical oleopurein, which inhibits viral replication and stimulates immune activity.

  Medicinal benefits: Common cold, flu, sinusitis, herpes, shingles, and general immune support. May also lower blood pressure and protect the cardiovascular system.

  Recommended dosage: 500–1,000 mg, three times daily.

  Cautions: None

- Elderberry (*Sambuccus nigra*)
  Description: Elderberry extract.
  History: Juice used to treat flus.
  Parts used: Berries
  Known active constituents: Unknown
  Actions: Prevents virus from penetrating cell walls.
  Medicinal benefits: Mainly the flu; also the common cold, fever, and cough.
  Recommended dosage: As directed on container.
  Cautions: None

- Larix (*Larix occidentalis*)
  Description: Light cream-colored powder, after extraction from the western larch tree.
  History: Developed in the last decade.
  Parts used: Tree bark
  Known active ingredients: Arabinogalactan—a type of polysaccharide.
  Actions: Enhances immune system activity.
  Medicinal benefits: Prevents and treats colds, infections, asthma, candida, and allergies.
  Recommended dose: As directed on container.
  Cautions: None

Chapter 4
DIGESTION AND DETOXIFICATION

~~~~~~

What are toxins?
How do toxins harm the immune system?
What natural therapies fight toxins?
Why is the liver so valuable?
What's leaky gut syndrome?
How can I improve my digestion?

Every day, we encounter an all-out assault by toxins. They taint the air we breathe, the food we eat, and the water we drink. Since the dawn of the industrial revolution more than a century ago, our environment has been exposed to tens of thousands of toxic chemicals. And that's just the ones we know about! Experts believe there are other still-unidentified toxins for which we don't know the long-term consequences. Inside our bodies, there are also toxins that form in the digestive tract. With this constant bombardment, it's no wonder why so many people are feeling the effects of "toxin overload."

This much we do know: People are exposed to more than 70,000 toxic chemicals. In fact, more than 20,000 toxic agents have been identified and linked to cancer, according to research by Patrick Quillin, author of *Beating Cancer with Nutrition*.[1]

Let's look at a snapshot of recent history. Between 1987 and 1994, officials from the U.S. Environmental Protection Agency required companies to report the amounts of environmental toxins they had released. The reported total: 111 million pounds!

NATURE'S VIRUS KILLERS

Here's the breakdown of where the toxins were released:

Source	Amount of toxins reported
Land	4 million pounds
Surface water	25 million pounds
Air	42 million pounds
Deep well water	40 million pounds

As staggering as 111 million pounds seems, that's only scratching the surface. EPA experts, concerned that companies are not reporting completely, estimated that the actual figure hovers around 2.2 *billion* pounds during that time period![2]

No one can escape all toxins, and I'm not recommending that you live underground or inside a plastic bubble. But knowledge, as the popular adage goes, is power. This chapter will arm you with important information to help you identify the major toxins, how they affect your body's key organs, and how you can better defend yourself and live a healthier life. In this effort to rid your body of these nasty chemicals, digestion plays a very vital role. That's why I've devoted the balance of this chapter to addressing common digestive problems. You will learn how your digestion system works and strategies to enhance your ability to break down foods.

When my patients ask what the best ways to strengthen their immune system are, I always emphasize the importance of good digestion and detoxification. The two go hand in hand. Without an efficient digestive system, toxins can accumulate in your body and tax not only your digestive system, but also your immune system. Over time, these systems can become so overwhelmed and overpowered that they become dysfunctional. Only by properly cleansing and purifying your body's cells can you truly achieve a healthy immune system and optimal vitality.

Let me illustrate by sharing a story involving one of my patients. Terri always seemed to "catch" the latest bug that was going around. She made repeated trips to conventional doctors who were unable to identify the cause of her condition. When Terri came to see me, she was sick and tired of, well, being sick and tired! In addition to her susceptibility to infections, she had a chronic skin rash on her back and suffered from fatigue.

I conducted a detoxification panel on Terri. This test is available from nutrition-oriented doctors. It requires the patient to ingest caffeine as well as aspirin and acetaminophen. Urine and saliva samples are then taken for analysis. The resulting profile shows how the liver and metabolic detoxification pathways are working. We discovered that Terri's liver was not detoxifying efficiently. I put Terri on a detoxification program that included a diet of fresh steamed vegetables, broths, herbs such as milk thistle and dandelion root for liver cleansing, and supplements specific to detoxification (explained later in the chapter). After two weeks Terri felt like a new person. Her energy levels were elevated, her skin cleared, and she was no longer prone to infections, even though she took no immunity-boosting supplements.

The premise of good health through detoxification is nothing new. It's been around for centuries. In Europe, mainstream medicine incorporates detoxification clinics and health spas as part of regular health-care plans. What is new is that more and more traditional physicians in North America are recognizing the value of detoxification, a concept that has always been embraced by naturopathic doctors and other holistic health-care practitioners.

Common Toxins: Metals, Pesticides, Herbicides, Digestive

We pay a price for progress. In the past 40 years industrial and manufacturing processes have greatly increased our exposure to toxic metals. The harmful effects of these metals vary depending on how much—and how often—people were exposed, their health status and age, and their detoxification abilities. Studies have shown that serious medical conditions, including kidney disease, high blood pressure, neurological disease, and cancer, are linked to exposure to toxic metals. These metals also cause damage to the DNA of cells (the genetic code), interfere with normal enzymatic processes, and lead to various mineral deficiencies. It is important to identify damaging toxic metals, remove (or at least lessen) the source, and bind these harmful substances so they can be "pulled out" of the body. Many experts feel the first line of treatment in a detoxification program is to identify and remove toxic metals. This takes a burden off the immune system. Alarmingly, it has been estimated by many nutritional experts, such as Dr. Passwater, that approximately one in every four people have heavy-metal toxicity to some degree.[3] Depending on the extent of heavy-metal toxicity diagnosed by your physician, specific treatments to remove these toxins can be recommended. For example, supplements such as N-acetylcysteine and vitamin C are helpful in removing mercury. For more serious cases chelation therapy is very helpful. This form of intravenous therapy uses the chemical EDTA to bind and help excrete heavy metals like lead. This is available only from physicians trained in chelation therapy.

What follows are some of the main metal toxins we face.

ALUMINUM

Aluminum is the most prevalent heavy metal in the earth's crust. Underground, aluminum is no health threat because it is inert and unable to be absorbed by the body. The real dangerous sources for aluminum are in our kitchens and medicine cabinets. People get exposed to this metal toxin from using aluminum cookware (pots and pans) and certain medicines that contain aluminum, such as antacids. In certain regions, the water supply can be contaminated with aluminum. Finally, let's not overlook aluminum's presence in antiperspirants, foil wrap, and soda-pop cans.

Aluminum is quite toxic to the nervous system and can cause problems with memory, balance, seizures, and neurological degenerative conditions. This metal encourages free radicals to damage the nervous tissue in the brain.

Occupational hazards can lead to aluminum contamination. A neurological study of 25 employees at an aluminum-smelting plant indicated that of these workers:

DIGESTION AND DETOXIFICATION

- *89 percent said they felt depressed*
- *88 percent reported they lost their balance often*
- *84 percent experienced memory loss*
- *84 percent experienced lack of coordination; and*
- *75 percent displayed mild impairment on memory tests.*

Researchers discovered that the level of health problems had a direct correlation to the amounts of exposure these workers had to aluminum in their jobs.[4]

LEAD

One of the sneakier heavy-metal toxins we encounter is lead. People accumulate lead slowly over time. This eventually harms vital organs like the brain as well as nerves and bones. Research has linked lead exposure to learning and behavior disorders in children. Adults who don't have enough calcium in their diets are also prone to lead toxins.

Compared to our cavemen ancestors, we, on average, have 100 to 1,000 times more lead in our bodies. Sure, we've taken some steps in the right direction, like eliminating lead from gasoline, but no amount of lead exposure is really safe.

Even though we've deleted lead from our car fuels, lead can still be found in water pipes in the home and workplace, and in air pollution, paint, batteries, and cigarette smoke.[5]

Lead toxicity can cause high blood pressure and atherosclerosis (hardening of the arteries) as well as neurological conditions such as tremors and anemia. If you need another reason to stop smoking (or to never start), scientists have discovered that smokers have twice the amount of lead in their bodies, on average, compared to non-smokers.

MERCURY

Mercury is a dangerous toxin to the body, especially to the nerves. So, what's the main source of mercury exposure? Just look inside your mouth. Mercury toxicity is primarily acquired through amalgam fillings. Mercury vapors are released over time

65

from amalgam fillings. Something as seemingly innocent as chewing gum (even sugar-free brands) accelerates this process because of the mechanics of the movement involved.

Even if you have mercury toxicity, you may not necessarily display any outward symptoms. A study was conducted involving 101 university students. Fifty had cavities treated with amalgam filling, 51 had no fillings in their mouths. The group with mercury fillings had a mercury concentration 26 percent higher in their hair and 201 percent higher in their urine than students with no fillings. Students who had their amalgam fillings later replaced with plastic and ceramic alternatives experienced improvements in mental and physical symptoms.[6]

Mercury is absorbed into the bloodstream and is stored in body tissues such as the brain, kidneys, and digestive tract. Mercury toxicity is implicated in many conditions, including neurological diseases such as multiple sclerosis, kidney disease, memory and learning problems, high blood pressure, cardiovascular disease, and various autoimmune conditions.

Other toxic elements that can be harmful to the immune system and organs of the body include antimony, arsenic, barium, cadmium, nickel, and uranium.

Symptoms of High Levels of Metal Toxicity

Metal	Symptoms
Aluminum	Appetite loss, imbalance, muscle aches, general feeling of weakness, kidney damage, psychosis, liver dysfunction, dementia.
Lead	Appetite loss, headaches, fatigue, dizziness, lack of coordination, memory problems, lack of concentration, irritability, muscle pain, stomach pain, anemia, indigestion, depression.
Mercury	Appetite loss, headaches, hearing loss, fatigue, lack of coordination, memory problems, numbness, vision problems, metallic taste, general weakness, anemia, hypertension, irritability, depression, instability.

Pesticides and Herbicides

Every year in the United States, more than one billion pounds of pesticides and herbicides are sprayed on crops. These chemicals have been linked to cancers, birth defects, and a host of neurological conditions. The chemicals accumulate in the body over time. I believe they contribute to a weak immune system. Special cleaning solutions may have a minor effect in washing off toxic residue. Therefore, I recommend the use of certified organic foods whenever possible. These foods, as indicated by their labels, are free of pesticides, herbicides, and any toxic fertilizer.

DIGESTIVE TOXINS

So far, we've identified the outside culprits. But it may surprise you to learn that we also produce a lot of our own toxins. This is known as "autointoxication," which refers to toxins formed in our own body. This occurs in our digestive tract, particularly in the small intestine and colon. When we do not break food down properly, especially proteins, toxic metabolites can be formed that get absorbed into the bloodstream. These metabolites poison our detoxification organs and immune system. Many different conditions can trigger this self-intoxication. Constipation, for example, can lead to the absorption of toxins.

The traditional naturopathic theory (which was disregarded by conventional physicians until recently) held that toxins are reabsorbed from the colon into the bloodstream. This theory has been proven conclusively in the past five years. This is a major reason why regular bowel movements are so important to your overall health.

So, how do you know if you have unhealthy levels of toxins in your body? Here are some common symptoms:

- *Acne*
- *Bad breath*
- *Chronic fatigue*

- *Frequent headaches*
- *Breast and colon cancer*
- *Nasty smelling stools*
- *Garlic intolerance*
- *Irritable bowel syndrome*
- *Chronic skin rashes*

Now that you have identified the enemy, let me explain your key allies in winning this detoxification war.

How the body detoxifies

Detoxification is critical to your survival. Fortunately, many of your organs are designed to metabolize and excrete toxins. Toxins are generally broken down in the liver, intestines, and kidneys. These toxins are mainly excreted out via the feces or urine. Two other organs, the lungs and skin (your largest organ), also help eliminate toxins through exhalation and perspiration.

Toxins that don't get the heave-ho tend to be deposited in body tissues, typically in fat tissue.

THE AMAZING LIVER

When ranking the importance organs that detoxify, the liver is like a five-star general. In a single second, thousands of enzymatic reactions take place inside your liver.

The liver must tackle toxins from within the body (autointoxication) and all toxins from the environment. The point is simple: you need a healthy liver to properly detoxify. The liver juggles many jobs. It filters nearly two quarts of blood every minute. This process helps filter out bacteria, antigen-antibody complexes, and other toxic substances. The liver produces about a quart of bile every day. Bile is necessary to help break down fats and absorb fat-soluble vitamins. Finally, the liver acts as a major transporter of toxins through the digestive tract and out through the stool.

Two basic phases of detoxification occur in the liver. During Phase 1, specialized cells in the liver, called the cytochrome

P450 system, neutralize a toxin or break it down to be excreted. The more stubborn toxins are sent to Phase 2's team of purifiers.

Some toxins may also be formed into free "intermediates," (substances that have been altered, making them easier to metabolize and excrete). If these intermediates cannot be broken down by Phase 2 detoxification, then free radicals are produced and can damage the liver and other parts of the body.

During Phase 2, the liver binds and deactivates toxins so that they can be excreted in the urine or carried by the bile into the stool for elimination. Many different vitamins and minerals, as well as amino acids, are required for Phase 2 detoxification.

Below I've identified the key ones, and provided toxin-fighting dosages that are safe for adults:

Detoxifier	Daily Dosage for Adults
Carotenoids	25,000 international units (IUs)
Vitamin C	1,000 to 5,000 mg
Vitamin E	400 to 800 IUs
Vitamin B-complex	100 mg
Magnesium	500 to 1,000 mg
Zinc	30 to 60 mg
Glutathione	1,000 to 3,000 mg
Glycine	1,000 mg
Alphalipoic Acid	100 mg daily

Specific herbs also promote proper liver health. At the top of my list is milk thistle. It contains an active constituent called silymarin, which protects the liver cells from being damaged and stimulates the regeneration of liver cells.[7] I typically recommend 150 mg taken three times daily of an 85-percent silymarin standardized extract of milk thistle. Additional herbs also help cleanse the liver:

Herb	Daily Dosage for Adults
Dandelion root	30 drops of tincture 3 times daily, or 500 mg capsules taken 3 times daily
Chicory root	30 drops of tincture 3 times daily, or 500 mg capsules taken 3 times daily
Chelidonium	30 drops of tincture 3 times daily, or 500 mg capsules taken 3 times daily
Globe artichoke	30 drops of tincture 3 times daily, or 500 mg capsules taken 3 times daily

Hair analysis

There is an easy, pain-free way to determine the levels of toxins in your body. The best screening method is hair analysis. It is an accurate and cost-effective way to assess heavy-metal exposure, as well as to check specific mineral values.

Hair values reflect the accumulation of heavy matals levels over time. Hair follicles have a rich supply of blood. Toxic elements circulate through the blood and are accumulated in the hair as it grows. They go through a process of hardening, whereby toxic metals are trapped. Confirmation of high levels of toxic metals can be confirmed with urine or blood measurements. Work with your natural health-care practitioner to identify these toxic metals.

Various labs specialize in hair and other metabolic tests. The one I use is called the Great Smokies Diagnostic Laboratory, in Asheville, North Carolina. For more information, go to their Web site at www.gsdl.com. In most cases, results are available within one to two weeks.

Detoxification Programs

To be your healthiest, you should practice detoxification daily. This includes whole, organic foods; drinking plenty of purified water and fresh juices; and exercising. Fasting can also be cleansing.

Too often, however, I see people participate in detoxification programs for a few days and then go back to their unhealthy lifestyle. This bouncing back and forth from good to bad can be very harmful. I equate it to yo-yo dieting. The constant shedding and then adding of pounds takes a toll on your body. So does going on—and then off—detoxification programs.

One of the easiest ways to detoxify is by fasting for a few days. People in good health can easily cleanse their bodies of excess toxins, without taxing their systems, by drinking plenty of purified water and/or juices. Don't worry; you won't starve. It actually takes several weeks to reach the starvation stage.

However, if you have a pre-existing medical condition, such as heart disease or diabetes, fast only under the supervision of a naturopathic physician or health-care practitioner. Otherwise, you could compound your problems. If toxins are released too quickly, your liver doesn't have time to metabolize them. This could harm your liver and other organs through the onslaught of free radicals. And, if you are already deficient in certain vitamins, minerals, amino acids, and phytochemicals, your body won't have the ammunition necessary to metabolize toxins during Phase 1 or 2.

Besides fasting, you could take supplements such as milk thistle, chlorophyll, amino acids, phytochemicals such as d-glucarate, sulphoraphane, and indole 3 Carbinol, as well as antioxidants. For best results, consult with a natural health-care practitioner who can customize a detoxification program that best meets your needs. For more information on detoxification, I highly recommend a book by naturopathic doctors Peter Bennett and Stephen Barrie called *7-Day Detox Miracle* (Prima Publishing).

Digestion

Paying attention to the types of foods we eat (and how they are processed) affects whether or not we develop digestive problems. Eating poorly makes it more difficult to break apart food, extract nutrients, and make sure nutrients are properly absorbed by the body.

Beyond eating habits, age also influences how well our digestive system performs. The older we get, the greater the chance that our appetite will decrease, our taste buds will become impaired, and our stomach will secrete less hydrochloric acid. Stress also impairs digestive function. Blood flow through the liver can also be reduced. The bottom line: less availability of nutrients being absorbed.

There are several conditions that affect how well the digestive system operates. Among the major ones are "leaky gut" syndrome, food allergies, parasites, and dysbiosis.

Leaky gut syndrome

Only now are many conventional physicians becoming aware of a common digestive condition well-known by naturopaths—"leaky gut syndrome." This occurs when the intestines become damaged from various causes (see below), resulting in them becoming more permeable. This allows larger-than-normal-sized molecules, especially proteins and pathogens, to be absorbed into the bloodstream. This then triggers the immune cells to attack these foreign particles. As a consequence, medical conditions, including food allergies and rheumatoid arthritis, may develop. The immune system gets depleted.

FACTORS CONTRIBUTING TO LEAKY GUT SYNDROME
- *Stress*
- *Use of medications such as nonsteroidal anti-inflammatory drugs, steroids, aspirin, and antibiotics*
- *Alcohol consumption*
- *Exposure to xenobiotics (chemicals foreign to the human body that are found in the food chain or water, including food additives, environmental pollutants, pesticides, and herbicides)*
- *Impaired digestion, leading to irritation and inflammation of the intestinal mucosa*
- *Food sensitivities*
- Yeast parasite infections
- Flora imbalance (balance between good and bad bacteria)

There are tests your holistic physician can conduct to see if you have leaky gut syndrome. These include the lactulose/mannitol absorption test. In this test a patient swallows two different-sized sugar molecules in a liquid solution. Lactulose is a large molecule and should not be absorbed to any great extent. Mannitol, a smaller sugar, is readily absorbed. If a higher than normal amount of lactulose shows up in the urine, then leaky gut syndrome is present.

Food allergies

Food allergies trigger digestion problems. An undiagnosed reaction can also wear down the immune system. If you eat a food you are sensitive to, your immune system will go to work reacting to it. As a result, there will be fewer "body soldiers" available to attack pathogens like viruses.

Nutrition-oriented physicians test their patients for food allergies. Identifying—and eliminating—food allergies has a beneficial domino effect on the rest of the body. The immune system is free to fight battles elsewhere. Many disorders influenced by digestive disorders, including eczema, rheumatoid arthritis, leaky gut, and many other chronic conditions, subside.

Common food allergies include dairy products, wheat, sugar, chocolate, citrus fruit, soy, and nuts. But keep in mind that every person is different. One person may be allergic to peanuts. Another may be allergic to chocolate *and* wheat. So, how can you tell what's causing your allergic reaction? You need to play food detective.

Determine what you ate—recently, over the past several days. Write each food down. Look at the list for foods that you suspect may be causing allergic reactions. Then, eliminate one of these foods for several days and see if any reactions occur. By doing this, one food at a time, you can pinpoint the true culprit.

Your natural health-care practitioner can help you identify your food reactions and help desensitize you to them.

Parasites

Parasites are opportunistic microbes that can invade the digestive tract. Once inside, they reek havoc. They cause a host of symptoms, ranging from diarrhea, bloating, and abdominal pain to fatigue. At the same time, they impair the immune system.

Some parasites, including giardia, hide inside the digestive tract for years without causing major symptoms. Everyone is susceptible to parasites, but the risks increase for people who travel outside North America and who have compromised immune system conditions such as HIV. The presence of parasites can be determined based on multiple stool sample analyses by labs that specialize in stool analysis.

You can fight parasites naturally with these safe and effective herbs:

Herb	Daily Dosage for Adults
Wormwood	20–30 drops or 500 mg, three times daily
Garlic	1 clove daily, or a 400 mg supplemental extract
Black walnut	20–30 drops or 500 mg, three times daily
Goldenseal	30 drops or 500 mg, three times daily
Barberry	30 drops or 500 mg, three times daily
Oregon grape root	30 drops or 500 mg, three times daily

In addition to these individual herbs, many effective Chinese herbal formulas for parasitic infections can be obtained from practitioners of Chinese herbal therapy.

Dysbiosis

The final major condition I'll address that harms the digestive system is dysbiosis. This term refers to flora imbalances in gut that lead to disease. Within the colon, and to a lesser extent the mouth, respiratory tract, and vaginal tract, are numerous species of microorganisms often referred to as flora. When they are in balance, they co-exist peacefully.

Lactobacilli and bifidobacteria are known as "friendly" bacteria. They help synthesize certain vitamins, metabolize hormones, and keep potentially harmful bugs (such as yeast) in check. When supplies of these "friendly" bacteria become depleted, yeast and other opportunistic pathogens take over. As a result, you get sick.

Most people are surprised to learn that antibiotics are one of the leading causes of dysbiosis. Prolonged and chronic use of antibiotics often leads to an overgrowth of yeast and other organisms in the digestive tract and other areas of the body. These organisms also produce their own toxic metabolites, which further burden the nervous system, liver, and immune system.

Besides antibiotics, intestinal dysbiosis can also be caused by poor diet (high sugar, low fiber, high fat, alcohol abuse), stress, poor digestive function, and environmental pollutants.

So, what can you do? Start eating yogurt. Not just any yogurt. Read the label and pick only brands containing live cultures. Yogurt's ingredients help replenish your supply of lactobacilli and other "friendly" flora in the body.

In addition, consider taking supplements that contain lactobacillus and other beneficial bacteria for several months to build up a natural army against harmful organisms.

Fiber, which I will discuss in more depth in the Chapter five, also plays a vital role as a fuel source for beneficial bacteria. So does a specific type of carbohydrate known as fructooligosaccharides (FOS). You can get plenty of FOS by eating asparagus, bananas, onions, and maple syrup. FOS is also one of the ingredients found in many flora supplements. It acts as a fuel source for beneficial bacteria such as lactobacilli.

Overall Digestion Aid

Natural medicine offers many different ways to improve digestive function. Herbs and plant enzymes lead the list.

To stimulate digestion and improve absorption of nutrients, rely on these herbs:

Herb	Activity	Daily Dosage for Adults
Gentian root	Releases bile, produces stomach acid	500 mg capsule, or 20 to 30 drops of tincture with every meal
Dandelion root	Secretes stomach acid, aids bile production and release	500 mg capsule, or 20 to 30 drops of tincture with every meal
Ginger root	Aids pancreatic enzymes, acts as anti-inflammatory in digestive tract	500 mg capsule, or 20 to 30 drops of tincture with every meal; sip cup of ginger root tea as needed.
Chamomile	Reduces intestinal gas	500 mg capsule, or 20 to 30 drops of tincture with every meal; sip cup of chamomile tea as needed
Peppermint tea	Reduces intestinal gas	Sip cup of peppermint tea as needed or take as an enteric-coated capsule or as a tincture

Plant enzymes are another natural booster. They are quite helpful to my patients. These enzymes are derived from plants and help support the pancreas's supply of enzymes in breaking down all foodstuffs. Generally, I recommend that my patients take two plant-enzyme capsules with each meal. Plant enzymes are available at health food stores and pharmacies, usually under the heading "Enzymes" in the natural health section. When reading the label, make sure the product contains proteases (protein enzymes), amylases (starch), and lipase (fats).

Homeopathy and acupuncture are the final natural therapies proven to improve digestion. They are addressed in detail in Chapter 9.

Chapter 5

NUTRITION: SUPER-CHARGE WITH FOOD

~~~~~~

What are the benefits of a plant-based diet?
Why are phytochemicals so vital?
What are my best food choices?
What are some good fats to eat?
What are the advantages of eating organic foods?

Let food be thy medicine, and medicine thy food.
—HIPPOCRATES, CIRCA 400 B.C.

Now, some 2,400 years later, the wise words of Hippocrates, the ancient Greek physician known as the Father of Medicine, remain a valuable reminder that foods keep us healthy and vitalize our immune system.

Even today, medical experts share Hippocrates' views of the importance of proper nutrition in the prevention—and treatment—of diseases. Poor nutrition has the opposite impact—creating and worsening disease.

Certainly supplements and herbs improve the efficiency of your immune system, but food is the stronger soldier in the battle against viruses. Eating the right foods fortifies your immune system with a fighting force of important nutrients and phytochemicals. Yes, you are what you eat. The choice is yours.

The best part is that it is easier to achieve sound nutrition than you may imagine. I'm not suggesting that you radically alter your eating habits—rather, fine-tune them so that your

77

body operates at its best. Even officials from the supplement industry recognize the benefits of consuming whole foods. In fact, they are moving toward the development of "whole food" extract products.

In this important chapter, I will help you gain insight into good and bad food choices. I will also offer practical ways to get more "nutritional mileage" out of the foods you eat, without adding calories.

Benefits of a Plant-Based Diet

Think green—especially at meal times. Diets dominated with plant-based foods have served as the cornerstone of health for many cultures throughout the ages. They will always form the necessary foundation for nutritious diets. Plants not only contain healing constituents such as vitamins, minerals, amino acids, enzymes, and phytonutrients, but they are low in harmful substances found in red meat and animal products, including saturated fat.

This is not to say I advocate that everyone convert to vegetarianism starting tomorrow. In fact, it may surprise you that I am not a vegetarian. What I am saying is that the majority of your foods should be plant-based. That means loading up more on fresh vegetables, fruits, grains, legumes, nuts, seeds and and reducing your intake of meats and animal products. You may even save money.

I often hear people complain about the number of supplements they need to take in order to feel good.

Consuming the right foods means spending less money on supplements to offset poor eating habits. Intensive studies on the American diet reveal that a large percentage of people choose foods that lack much nutritional value. The burgers-and-fries bunch greatly outnumbers the fruits-and-vegetables group. Alarmingly, nearly seven out of ten American adults surveyed in one study admitted that they rarely—if ever—eat fruits and vegetables rich in vitamins A and C.[1]

One of the under-rated aspects of plant foods is fiber. This indigestible portion of plants serves many beneficial functions.

Fiber helps to prevent the absorption of fats, toxins, and excess cholesterol into the body. It also helps to slow the release of blood sugar into the bloodstream, making for more balanced blood sugar levels. Fiber, when paired with water, helps keep bowels function properly. Finally, fiber assists in replenishing good bacteria in the digestive tract.

The sources of fiber fall into two main groups: soluble and insoluble. Soluble fibers lower blood cholesterol, balances glucose levels and improve elimination through the intestines. Soluble fibers dissolve in water and bind cholesterol and fats. Insoluble fibers speed gastrointestinal digestion, increase bowel weight, slow down the absorption of glucose into the blood, and slow starch breakdown. Insoluble fibers do not dissolve or break down in the digestive system, so they help form the bulk of stools and bind toxins (like a cowboy rounding up a herd of cattle) to be excreted.

In general, soluble fibers tend to be found in fruits, legumes, barley, and oats. Insoluble fibers are often found in wheat, cereals, and vegetables.

SOLUBLE FIBER FOODS
Apples
Bananas
Kiwis
Oranges
Black beans
Black-eyed peas
Kidney beans
Navy beans
Pinto beans
Barley
Grits
Oatmeal

INSOLUBLE FIBER FOODS
Whole wheat
Pumpernickel bread
Rye bread

Bran cereal
Bean sprouts
Broccoli
Brussel sprouts
Cabbage
Carrots
Cauliflower
Kale
Spinach
Sweet potatoes

FIBER GOAL: 40 TO 50 GRAMS DAILY

Power of Phytonutrients

Phytonutrients, also known as phytochemicals, are potent protectors of the body, particularly the immune system. These naturally occurring substances give plants their characteristic flavor, color, aroma, and resistance to disease. Nutritional experts have identified more than 4,000 phytonutrients from fruits, vegetables, legumes, nuts, and whole grains. Experts estimate thousands more are yet to be discovered. Given these large numbers, it's understandable why whole foods are so important to your overall health.[2]

Phytonutrients are also associated with the prevention and treatment of illnesses such as cancer, heart disease, diabetes, high blood pressure, and other common medical conditions. They help the immune system indirectly by aiding the cells in detoxification, which reduces the demand placed on the immune cells.

One of the most vital groups of phytonutrients is the carotenoid family. The star of this family is beta carotene. This one often grabs the medical spotlight in health books, magazines, newspapers, and radio and television broadcasts, but the entire carotenoid family is necessary for optimal health.

More than 600 types of carotenoids have been identified, making them the most abundant group of phytonutrients.

Besides the popular beta carotene (carrots are rich in this type) there are lesser-known but equally important carotenoids: alpha carotene, lutein, and lycopene. Carotenoids are among nature's most powerful antioxidants. They help to prevent free radical damage to the cells of the body.

High concentrations of carotenoids are found in dark green, red, yellow, and orange fruits and vegetables. The best food sources include carrots, pumpkins, red and yellow peppers, sweet potatoes, tomatoes, collard greens, and spinach.

Flavonoids are another big class of phytonutrients. Thousands have been identified. Common flavonoids you may have heard about include citrus bioflavonoids such as rutin, quercitin, and hesperedin. Other flavonoid-rich supplements include grape-seed extract, Pycnogenol, green tea, ginkgo biloba, artichoke extract, and milk thistle.

For flavonoids taken as supplements, I recommend:

- *Grape seed extract or Pycnogenol—50 to 150 mg daily*
- *Quercitin—500 to 1,500 mg daily*
- *Citrus bioflavonoids—1,000 to 3,000 mg daily*
- *Green tea–1 to 3 cups daily*

Flavonoids have demonstrated potent antioxidant activity. They are also helpful in reducing the risk of cancer. Flavonoids help prevent pathogens such as viruses from penetrating through the skin. They also support T-lymphocyte activity.

Excellent food sources of flavonoids include blueberries, tangerines, cherries, bilberries, citrus fruit, apples, peppers, onions, and carrots.

Let's take a closer look at specific food sources, specific phytochemicals, and how they benefit the body.

- **Citrus (oranges, lemons, limes, grapefruits)**
  Phytochemicals: carotenoids, flavonoids, D-limonene
  Benefits: carotenoids and flavonoids act as powerful antioxidants and improve circulation. D-limonene helps to detoxify cancerous toxins.

NATURE'S VIRUS KILLERS

- **Red grapes** (red wine)
  Phytochemicals: anthocyanadins, ellagic acid, resveratrol, quercitin
  Benefits: prevent cellular damage, keep blood thin, and reduce risk of heart disease and stroke.

- **Soy** (soy milk, tofu, soy protein, and others)
  Phytochemicals: isoflavonoids such as genistein, diadzein, saponins, lignans
  Benefits: balances estrogen levels; protects against breast, uterine, colon, and prostate cancer; reduces cholesterol; enhances antioxidant activity.

- **Tomatoes, red peppers, watermelon, grapefruit**
  Phytochemicals: carotenoids—mainly lycopene
  Benefits: reduce risk of prostate cancer; antioxidant activity.

- **Whole grains** (whole wheat, barley, oats, rye)
  Phytochemicals: phytoestrogens, saponins, terpenoids, phytic acid, ellagic acid
  Benefits: bind cancerous toxins.

- **Tea** (green, black)
  Phytochemicals: flavonoids, such as catechins
  Benefits: potent antioxidants; promotes cellular detoxification; prevents cancer and cardiovascular disease.

- **Nuts** (almonds, cashews, walnuts, chestnuts)
  Phytochemicals: saponins, ellagic acid
  Benefits: cardiovascular protection.

- **Herbs and spices** (sage, rosemary, thyme, oregano, ginger, and others)
  Phytochemicals: various
  Benefits: potent antioxidants and cancer protection.

- **Flax** (seeds and flour)
  Phytochemicals: lignans
  Benefits: cancer protection.

- **Cruciferous vegetables** (broccoli, broccoli sprouts, cauliflower, brussel sprouts, cabbage, kale)
  Phytochemicals: indole, isothiocyanates-sulphoraphane, carotenoids
  Benefits: anti-cancer; detoxification; immune system supporter.

Green Drinks—The Next Best Choice

Yes, you can drink your vegetables. If diving into a plate of lima beans or brussel sprouts doesn't stimulate your appetite, I offer this healthy alternative: green drinks.

Green drinks are popular supplements endorsed by health food experts, including me. Green drinks are my favorite beverages. The term "green drink" comes from the fact that most of these supplements are high in green plant foods such as barley grass, wheat grass, alfalfa, chlorella, spirulina, and other plant materials. They all contain a rich supply of chlorophyll, which is nature's great cellular detoxifier and rejuvenator. Many of the green drinks also contain detoxifying herbs such as milk thistle and dandelion root. Green tea is also and excellent choice.

So, if you're not a big vegetable eater and you realize vegetables and fruits are rich sources of phytochemicals, I recommend you try green drinks. They act as an insurance policy for your body, supplementing these valuable nutrients. By doing so, you are taking a valuable step toward maintaining a strong immune system and preventing infectious diseases and some types of cancers.

So, how do they taste? Many people mix green drinks with water or fruit juices like apple juice. Pick what tastes best for you. Some formulas also contain natural sweeteners such as mango juice and stevia. Finally, whole food concentrates are also available in capsules.

Immune-Boosting Culinary Herbs and Spices

The fresh clove of garlic. The big yellow onion in the pantry. The fresh leaves of basil, cilantro, and parsley. All of these herbs and spices make dishes in the kitchen come alive with aroma and taste. They also provide beneficial effects to your immune system.

Let's take a closer look at a few of these healing herbs and spices.

Garlic. Many viruses are inhibited by garlic. These include herpes simplex 1 (cold sores), herpes simplex 2 (genital herpes), human rhinovirus type 2 (cold), parainfluenza virus type 3, vaccinia virus, and vesicular stomatitis virus.[3] One of garlic's active ingredients is allicin, one of nature's most potent plant antiseptics. Garlic also contains many other therapeutic constituents.

Immune-Boosting Soup

Try this tasty recipe the next time a viral invader (such as a cold or flu virus) heads your way. All these ingredients are loaded with compounds that arm your immune system against a viral attack:

> 1 cup fresh burdock stems, chopped
> 5 cloves of garlic, minced
> 1 onion, diced
> 1/2 cup fresh okra, chopped
> 3 cups water
> A pinch of salt, pepper, and turmeric

In a large pot, add the water, burdock, onions, garlic, and okra. Bring to a boil, then reduce the heat and cover the pot with a lid. Allow the soup to simmer until the vegetables are soft. You can then season to taste, using salt, pepper, and turmeric, or one of your favorite spices. This recipe makes two servings.

Onions. Onions are loaded with antiviral and antibacterial agents. Ingredients in onions also help lower blood pressure and have antiworm effects.

Ginger. Ginger has a long medicinal history. This spice has been used on viral infections causing sore throats, colds, the flu, and intestinal infections since the days of ancient China. Ginger works especially well when you are chilled and need a warming herb. It also makes a great medicinal tea.

Fats that Heal and Fats that Steal

F-A-T. This little three-letter word is saddled with a bad reputation. Most people associate the word fat with a negative emotion. They think all fats will make them overweight.

The real skinny on fat is that we all need it in our diet to stay alive. But we need specific, healthy types of fat known as essential fatty acids. Much of the metabolism of the hormonal, immune, and cellular systems depend on these fatty acids: alpha linolenic (omega-3) and linoleic (omega-6) acids.

Most people get an imbalance between the omega-3 and omega-6 fatty acids by consuming too many omega-6 fatty acids and too few omega-3 foods. Many experts feel that a 4:1 ratio of omega-6 to omega-3 fatty acids is optimal for good health. However, according to experts such as Dr. Artemis P. Simopoulos in her book *The Omega Plan*, "The typical Western diet contains approximately fourteen to twenty times more omega-6 fatty acids than omega-3s."[4] The main reason for this imbalance is the omega-6s containing vegetable oils, which are so commonly used in cooking and processed foods. Oils such as safflower, corn, sunflower, and the others listed in the chart on page 86 are high in omega-6 fatty acids. People need to consume more of the omega-3 fatty acids found in fish (salmon, herring, halibut, trout), in nuts such as walnuts, in vegetables such as flaxseeds, and in beans, broccoli, barley, oats, lettuce, purslane, and seafood such as seaweed. Oils such as canola and flaxseed are good sources of omega-3 fatty acids.

Omega-3 oils	Omega-6 oils
Flaxseed oil	Safflower oil
Fish oil	Corn oil
Canola oil	Cottonseed oil
Walnut oil	Sunflower seed oil
Soybean oil	Soybean oil
	Sesame oil
	Peanut oil
	Borage oil
	Evening primrose oil
	Grape seed oil

An imbalance between omega-3 (too little) and omega-6 fatty acids leads to the activation of inflammatory pathways. This predisposes one to autoimmune conditions like rheumatoid arthritis and other inflammatory diseases. These inflammatory pathways also suppress the immune system, leading to an increased susceptibility to cancer and cardiovascular disease. Many practitioners recommend the intake of omega-3 fatty acid sources such as flaxseed oil to prevent and complement cancer treatments.

Harmful fats need to be eliminated from the diet. Topping the list of bad fats are the saturated ones. Saturated fats are semi-solid at room temperature. The same reaction occurs with saturated fat as with an imbalance of omega-6 and omega-3 fatty acids—that is, the creation of inflammatory and immune-suppressing reactions in the body. Saturated fats are found in dairy products, red meat, and pork.

Second on the bad-fat list are margarines, shortenings, and most hydrogenated vegetable oils. The process of hydrogenation (adding of a hydrogen molecule to an unsaturated fatty acid molecule to make oils into a solid) results in the formation of trans fatty acids. Trans fatty acids are harmful in that they interfere with the body's metabolism and use of helpful essential fatty acids. Margarine and other trans fatty acid sources increase LDL cholesterol (a harmful form of cholesterol associated with heart disease) and lower HDL cholesterol (a protective form of cholesterol).

One oil I have not mentioned is olive oil. Although it is low in omega-3 fatty acids, it is a good source of monounsaturated fatty acids, which promote cardiovascular health. Monounsaturated fats are more stable than other fats and do not generate free radicals as easily as other types of fats. Free radicals are unpaired electrons that travel around the body looking for another electron to pair up with. This can lead to the damage of DNA in cells. It can also lead to the oxidation of cholesterol, which is the real culprit when it comes to cholesterol and heart disease. Canola and olive oil are the best oils to incorporate into your diet.

Information on flaxseed appears never ending. In addition to being an excellent source of omega-3 fatty acids, it also contains valuable phytochemicals known as lignans. These lignans have been shown to have anticancer, antifungal, antibacterial, and antiviral activity.[5,6] Flaxseed can be ground up and added to salads or meals. I recommend eating a quarter cup a day as a good starting amount. Flaxseed oil is also a good option at one tablespoon daily. Look for brands that have a high lignan concentration. Other excellent supplemental sources of omega-3 fatty acids include salmon and tuna oil.

Avoiding the Sugar Trap

How sweet it *isn't*. Sugar is disguised everywhere in our food supply. It may surprise you to learn that the average North American eats over 150 grams of sugar daily and 125 pounds of sugar each year![7]

Simple sugars such as sucrose, glucose, and fructose are found in almost all the foods we eat. These sugars suppress the activity of immune cells, making us more prone to disease and infection. Studies have indicated the immune-suppressing effects of sugar. Ingestion of sugar by itself can lead to immune system depression thirty minutes after ingestion and can last up to five hours. A study found in the *American Journal of Clinical Nutrition* showed that a 50 percent reduction in neutrophil activity (this is significant, as neutrophils make up approximately 70 percent of total white blood cells) occured two hours after ingesting sugar . The white blood cells were suppressed for up to five hours after ingesting a sugar solution on an empty stomach.[8, 9]

One way to reduce the harmful effects of sugars is not to ingest them on an empty stomach. In other words, if you are going to have a fruit drink or sugary dessert, have it with a meal. Why? When combined with protein and fiber from vegetables, you can slow down the release of sugar into the bloodstream. By doing this, there will be less of a concentration of sugar in your blood to impact your immune cells.

Unfortunately, artificial sweeteners may behave like neuro-toxins, damaging your nervous system and possibly weakening your immune system. Even though the U.S. Food and Drug Administration has approved the use of saccharin, aspartame, and acesulfame potassium (acesulfame-K), I strongly urge my patients to stay clear of these products. Saccharin and aspartame are found in many diet soda drinks and fruit juice beverages. Acesulfame is found in many tabletop sweeteners, instant coffees, and desserts.

If you have a sweet tooth, there are healthier alternatives. My favorite natural sweeteners include the herb stevia and honey. Both can be added to juices and protein drinks. Although honey does contain simple sugars, it also has immune-enhancing and antimicrobial qualities, as well as minerals.

QUALITY PROTEIN SOURCES

The body needs quality protein sources for tissue repair and to form antibodies to assist immune cells. Quality protein sources include vegetables such as legumes, nuts, seeds, and grains. Animal sources include fresh fish, free-range poultry from these chickens, eggs, and organic dairy products, such as cheese, yogurt, and milk.

People with higher physical activity levels require higher amounts of protein for muscle repair.

The Value of Organic Foods

When choices are available, I recommend to all my patients that they pick fresh organic food which are grown without herbicides, pesticides, or other harmful synthetic chemicals. Organic foods are much safer than foods treated with these chemicals. Studies have shown that organic foods contain a higher mineral content than conventionally grown foods typically available at most supermarkets.[10] Foods containing preservatives and colorings can weaken an immune system over time. Yellow dye No. 5 (known as tartrazine) and red dyes are found in countless packaged foods. Preservatives such as sodium benzoate, nitrates, and sulfites are allergens for a lot of people. Nitrates and nitrites, found in hot dogs and cured meats, for example, have been shown to be cancer-causing agents, especially for stomach cancer and brain cancer.[11]

Yes, organic foods cost more, but isn't your health worth it?

The Importance of Drinking Quality Water

Good quality water is often one of the most underrated factors in ensuring a healthy diet. All waters are the same, right? Very wrong.

You need clean, filtered water to keep your immune system operating at its very best. Remember, water is the most abundant substance in the human body. So, we should be consuming the highest quality. Water helps our organs function properly, flushes out toxins, and bolsters our immune system.

Even if you rarely broke into a sweat in a day, you should still drink at least forty-eight ounces of pure, quality water each day. Finding quality water can be challenging. Most of the tap water supply is contaminated with pesticides and other chemicals such as PCBs, heavy metals (such as lead, chlorine, fluoride), or infectious organisms such as giardia and other parasites.

Quality among bottled water companies varies widely. Distilled water is not preferable because the important minerals are removed. The optimal water filtration system is one that uses a reverse osmosis unit, followed with a carbon filter. If possible, get one for your home for your drinking water.

Steer Clear of CATS

No, I'm not referring to those furry feline friends of ours. Rather, this is an acronym for four of the biggest health threats facing us today: Caffeine, Alcohol, Tobacco, and Sugar. Put them together, and they spell CATS.

NATURE'S VIRUS KILLERS

When you consume these substances beyond moderation, they become toxins in your body. You often hear coffee drinkers proclaim that caffeine gets them that needed jolt to start their day. But they pay a price for this temporary state of energy and stimulation. Over time, caffeine damages the immune system and other body systems, including the liver and the heart. Caffeine acts like a thief inside the body, robbing it of vitamin C, calcium, magnesium, chromium, B vitamins, and other essential vitamins and minerals.

Good news: There are some healthy alternatives to coffee that offer energy without the harmful side effects. Switch to herbal teas, especially green teas. They contain a rich source of antioxidants known as polyphenols. These teas also contain phytochemicals that aid the body in detoxification. Consider drinking teas made from fresh or dried leaves of chamomile, peppermint, and a wide variety of other great choices.

An occasional glass of red wine is actually healthy for one's heart, because it provides antioxidants. But drinking more than two glasses of any alcohol a day, even red wine, can spell trouble for your immune system and vital organs. Excessive amounts of alcohol act like poison in your body and deplete valuable minerals and vitamins (such as zinc, vitamin A, B vitamins, vitamin C, magnesium, and essential fatty acids). Alcohol also creates an imbalance in the intestinal floral, which serve a vital role in keeping the immune system healthy. I much prefer that my patients drink organic grape juice over red wine to prevent heart disease and maintain a healthy immune system.

In summary, making smart food—and drink—choices can make the difference in fighting off viral infections. As I've stressed during this chapter, I'm not asking you to suddenly eat only salads and give up the foods you crave. You can achieve balance.

Let me share with you the story of Carol.

Carol existed on what I term the "SAD" diet (the Standard American Diet). It generally consisted of fast foods, refined sugars, coffee, meat, and processed foods. Fresh fruits and vegetables ranked low on her food chain. Not surprisingly, she was constantly coming down with viral or bacterial pneumonia.

NUTRITION: SUPERCHARGE WITH FOOD

She came to see me for help. We made gradual changes in her diet. We began by having Carol add a salad to her fast-food meals at lunch and dinner. By adding this plant-based fare, her levels of vitamins, minerals, phytochemicals, and fiber all increased.

Then, we reduced the amount of coffee she drank—again, gradually. Over a period of one month, I was able to wean her from eight cups of coffee a day to three. As a healthy substitute, she started to drink one fresh vegetable or fruit juice (made in her home juicer) each day. She began drinking more herbal teas and less soda pop.

These two simple changes in her diet strengthened Carol's immune system enough so that pneumonia stopped being a problem for her.

Chapter 6
HORMONES: BODY GUARDS

~~~~~~

What role does the thymus gland play?
What is DHEA?
How does melatonin help the immune system?
How do growth hormones help the liver?

Hormones are powerful chemicals in the body that directly impact our moods, memory, energy levels, and how well we deal with the unavoidable: stress. Hormones are responsible for controlling blood pressure, sexual function, and growth. Often, medical conditions are a result of too little or too much secretion of one or more hormones.

Just as you pay attention to eating healthy foods, exercising regularly, and taking the appropriate supplements, so should you make sure your hormones are balanced and healthy. Collectively, all these factors help you maintain a super-strong immune system able to out-muscle viral invaders.

Headlining the list of immune-friendly hormones are

- *Thymus*
- *DHEA*
- *Melatonin*
- *Growth hormone*

Thymus Gland: The Virus Hunter

To a large extent, the thymus gland acts like the commander-in-chief for the immune-system army. The thymus is composed of two lobes that are located below the thyroid gland and behind the sternum (breastbone). This gland is very large at birth and is necessary to develop a child's immune system. But by age of fifty, the thymus gland has shrunk considerably and has little or no activity.

The role of the thymus is to mature T lymphocytes (T refers to the thymus). This is an important part of cell-mediated immunity, which I addressed in detail in Chapter 2. The culprit behind chronic infections is often impaired T-lymphocyte activity.

While residing in the thymus gland, T-lymphocytes become T-helper cells (also known as CD4 cells). They help the immune system recognize foreign invaders like viruses and bacteria. T-lymphocytes may also be converted into T Supressor cells. These cells keep the imune system in check and prevent it from going haywire. Their assistance is important to the body's defense against developing medical conditions, ranging from cancer and allergies to autoimmune conditions such as lupus and rheumatoid arthritis.

A healthy functioning thymus gland starts from day one, when an infant receives protection against infections through breast-feeding. Studies show that breast-fed infants, on average, experience fewer infections and allergies than formula-fed babies. Studies indicate that breast-fed infants actually have larger thymus glands compared to formula-fed infants. In fact, the thymus glands of breast-fed infants were more than twenty times bigger than those of formula-fed infants![1]

Several hormones secreted by the thymus gland help to regulate the immune system. I'll focus on what I consider to be the Super Five: thymosin, thymulin, thymic humoral factor, thymopoietin, and thymic protein A. All five hormones appear crucial to the proper functioning of the immune system. For example, thymic humoral factor appears to have specific antiviral effects, and thymic protein activates the T helper cells. The latter provides the immune system with a more efficient warning system for the T helper cells patrolling the body for unwanted intruders. Thymic proteins signal T killer cells to rush in and destroy these intruders.[2-4]

How can you tell if your thymus hormones are in top shape? Health-care practitioners pay attention to two criteria. First is the health history of the patient. Does this person catch infections easily and often? Once infected, does the condition linger? Does he or she have chronic infections such as hepatitis, herpes, or a deterioration of the immune system such as cancer? The second main requirement is answered when a holistic-minded physician performs blood tests to measure the levels of thymus hormones.

If the patient's history and/or blood tests indicate a thymus-deficiency, then extracts are indicted. Thymic protein A is available commercially in extract form for therapeutic use. Many doctors report significant benefits to the immune system when patients supplement thymic protein A. Another common form, found in health-food stores and used by nutrition-oriented practitioners, is a glandular extract from calf thymus. Glandular treatment is nothing new in medicine. Its premise is that the ingestion of glandular extract will strengthen and improve the functioning of the equivalent human gland.

Thymus glandular extract has been shown to be effective for immune-related disorders, such as reoccurring respiratory-tract infections in children, hepatitis B, low white blood cell counts in cancer patients undergoing chemotherapy treatments, allergies, and hay fever. It is interesting to note that thymus extracts have been shown to be effective in treating acute and chronic cases of viral hepatitis.[5, 6]

In addition, the use of thymus extract can be helpful for those with AIDS. It helps to improve T helper cell counts, which are necessary to fight life-threatening secondary infections affecting people with this condition.[7]

HOW TO USE THYMUS EXTRACTS

There is no standard dosage for thymus glandular extract. You should follow the dosage directions recommended by the specific manufacturer. However, I will offer you some helpful tips. First, choose only organic sources for thymus glandular extracts, to ensure quality and that the products are free from harmful pesticides and herbicides.

Rely on higher dosages to address acute infections and lower dosages to treat long-term immune support. You can take thymus extract with other supplements, such as immune-enhancing herbs, without any harmful consequences.

In addition, thymic protein A is now being used by many physicians, because it offers immune-modulating effects. As I mentioned, Thymic protein A is now available in supplemental form.

To guarantee optimal functioning of thymic hormones, I also recommend that you take vitamins C, E, B-complex (especially B-6), selenium, and beta-carotene supplements daily. These can be taken as part of a high-potency multivitamin.

For children, thymus extracts can be given safely as long as you give them amounts equivalent to one-fourth to one-half of an adult daily dose. Although there have been few studies done on them, other physicians and I have found thymus supplementation to be quite useful for children. There do not appear to be any side effects among children receiving thymus supplementation.

I have also found homeopathic preparations of thymus extract effective for both children and adults.

DHEA

One of the most well-accepted hormones to enter the marketplace is DHEA (dehydroepiandosterone). DHEA is touted as an antiaging hormone that helps fight the ravages of time and stress, including low energy, poor memory, high cholesterol, heart disease, and weight gain.

DHEA is one of the most studied hormones, with more than 5,000 research studies completed on it. DHEA is the most abundant steroid hormone in the body. It is produced mainly in the adrenal glands which are located at the top of each kidney. Adrenal glands produce and secrete stress hormones, including DHEA and cortisol, DHEA is also produced in smaller amounts by the brain and skin.

DHEA is often referred to as a fountain-of-youth hormone, as it serves as a precursor to many of the hormones in the body, including estrogen, progesterone, and testosterone. In general, levels of DHEA reach a peak value around age thirty, and then gradually decline in the subsequent decades. By keeping DHEA at youthful levels, you can maintain a virile immune system.

Many physicians feel that low levels of DHEA are associated with most major illnesses. Evidence suggests a direct correlation of low DHEA levels with immune deficiency syndromes such as cancer and AIDS. A study published in 1992 in the *Journal of Immunodeficiency* looked at men diagnosed with HIV virus and their levels of DHEA. This longitudinal study showed a relationship between low serum DHEA levels in HIV-infected men and a more rapid progression to AIDS.[8] DHEA improves the immune system's resistance to viral and bacterial infections. It also improves the rate of recovery from infections.

Studies suggest that DHEA may help prevent certain cancers. In one study by Gordon, et al., thirty-five people who eventually developed bladder cancer were compared to sixty-nine people in the control group. Pre-diagnosed levels of DHEA were substantially lower among the thirty-five than those in the control group. As the group of thirty-five developed cancer, their DHEA levels continued to plummet.[9]

Low levels of DHEA and other stress hormones, such as pregnenelone and cortisol, are often a result of chronic stress. Under acute stress, our adrenal glands produce higher amounts of DHEA to support metabolism and increase the immune system's resilience to stress. But under chronic stress, the adrenal glands' production of stress hormones slow down. This leads to the breakdown of many systems in the body, especially the immune system.

Levels of DHEA, along with other hormones, can be accurately tested by your physician. As a benchmark, women produce 19 mg of DHEA and men produce 31 mg of DHEA per day. One popular way of testing DHEA levels is through a salivary hormone analysis. One of the advantages of saliva over blood tests is that multiple samples can be taken throughout the day to give a clearer indication of levels. Also, saliva tests measure the amount of "free," or active hormone, unlike blood tests which look at "bound" or inactive hormone. And, you don't have to be jabbed by a needle! Based on these lab results, a person can safely take DHEA supplements to restore optimal levels. A physician should definitely monitor daily supplemental doses above 25 mg.

DHEA supplementation seems to enhance a person's resistance to viral infections and to increase the rate of recovery from infections.

Making lifestyle changes that relieve stress (such as taking up regular exercise and practicing relaxation techniques such as mental imagery) and increasing your intake of vitamin C can help increase DHEA levels naturally.

Melatonin

Most people have heard about the benefits of melatonin for insomnia and jet lag, but did you know that this hormone also has a powerful effect on the immune system? Melatonin is manufactured and secreted by the pineal gland, located in the brain. The pineal gland helps set and control your natural body clock.

Normally, melatonin is released at night to help you fall asleep. During the day, sunlight and artificial lighting suppresses melatonin.

Animal studies have shown that beyond helping you sleep, melatonin improves the size and function of the thymus gland. This indirectly improves the power of the immune system.

One interesting study done in 1991 by Irwin, et al., examined twenty-three men between the ages of twenty-two and sixty-one. These men were purposely deprived of sleep between 3 A.M. and 7 A.M. As expected, test results indicated they had below-normal melatonin levels. Lab tests also showed that there was a dramatic decrease in their white blood cell counts, especially in the natural killer cells that have antiviral effects. Dosages for melatonin typically range from 0.3 mg to 5 mg.[10]

Thyroid Hormone

Low thyroid function can make one susceptible to recurring infections. The thyroid hormone helps to control our body metabolism. An underfunctioning thyroid can weaken the immune system. In his book, *Hypothyroidism: The Unsuspected Illness* (Harper & Row), Dr. Broda Barnes states that approximately 40 percent of the population has a problem with low thyroid. I see this very common problem in my female patients over forty and with elderly patients. Blood tests are frequently ineffective in diagnosing low thyroid. Common symptoms, other than susceptibility to infections, include cold hands and feet, constipation, poor memory, dry skin, and an inability to lose weight. Taking one's temperature upon awakening three mornings in a row can give an accurate indication of thyroid function. Readings consistently below 97.6 degrees Fahrenheit signal low thyroid function. My preferred treatment, and of many of my holistically minded colleagues, is to use natural Armor Thyroid to bring thyroid levels back up to normal ranges.

Growth Hormone

Growth hormone is an incredibly powerful hormone that has many effects on the body. It is released by the pituitary gland. The levels of growth hormone peak in a person's twenties and then slowly decline. During childhood development growth hormone increases bone length and density, as well as muscle mass. Benefits of growth hormone supplementation for adults include: a stronger immune system; stronger, thicker bones; increased lean muscle mass; increased energy; increased sexual performance; improved heart function; lower cholesterol; and many others. Growth hormone must only be used under the guidance of a knowledgeable physician to avoid serious side effects caused by overdoses.

In summary, hormones that are in balance and in harmony play a vital role in ensuring a strong immune system. Although I have highlighted the values of thymic hormones, DHEA, melatonin thyroid, and growth hormones, I cannot underscore enough that all hormones work in harmony together for optimal health. An imbalance in just one hormone can trigger a cascade effect and throw off the balance of other hormones.

I recommend that you seek the guidance of a physician knowledgeable in hormone therapy to learn more about the balance between your hormones. Your conventional medical doctor can order blood tests that measure these hormones. Even better, look for a physician who measures these hormones by salivary analysis. Many physicians, including me, believe it is more accurate than blood tests and will become the preferred method of hormone analysis in the future.

Chapter 7
VITAMINS AND MINERALS: ANTIVIRAL AGENTS

~~~~~~

Why take supplements?
How do supplements fortify the immune system?
Which vitamins and minerals are most essential?

Even the most health-conscious person can't rely on nutritious food alone to maintain a strong, virus-resistant body. Maybe you've even tried faithfully to follow the U.S. Recommended Daily Allowances by eating two to three servings of fruits, three to five servings of vegetables, and six to eleven servings of grains every day. You probably discovered quickly how good intentions can be overrun by the demands of daily life.

Face it: We live hectic, on-the-go lives in which we don't always eat the right foods. That meal of a hamburger and french fries is justified as a time-saver as we dash from here to there. That ice cream sundae is regarded as well-spent bonding time with our child or grandchild. Or, we oversleep and skip breakfast.

Now more than ever, we need vitamin and mineral supplements to make up for nutrients lacking in our diets. In fact, supplements do more than simply overcome nutritional shortfalls. Scientific research indicates that certain key supplements can make you healthier by keeping your immune system operating at its very best.

Supplements also provide you with large amounts of essential vitamins and minerals that would be nearly impossible to obtain by eating food alone. Let's say you want to stave off a cold. You look for a food source loaded in vitamin C, known to boost immune systems and duel viruses. One orange contains about 70 mg of vitamin C. But in order to fortify your immune system against cold viruses, you would need to take about 3,000 mg of vitamin C daily. That translates into eating forty-two oranges a day!

The example of the orange-for-colds illustrates the vital role that vitamins and mineral supplements play in our lives today. This chapter will explore how supplements work and which ones you should focus on for specific viral conditions. I've provided information on scientific studies that validate the need for supplements. I've also given you recommended intakes based on age.

Please let me re-emphasize that the road to good health starts with a good diet. I've outlined some nutritional strategies in Chapter 5. In addition to the vitamins and minerals I've spotlighted in this chapter, I also encourage you to take a high potency multivitamin without iron (unless you have been diagnosed with iron-deficiency anemia).

Supplements and Your Immune System

Your immune system requires a host of vitamins and minerals to function optimally. As mentioned earlier, even the healthiest eaters among us are often deficient in one or more important nutrients.

In a recent scientific study, nearly 12,000 American adults were polled about their eating habits. They were questioned about what they ate during a typical twenty-four-hour period.

The results indicated that

- *41 percent did not eat any fruit,*
- *72 percent did not eat any fruits or vegetables rich in vitamin C,*
- *80 percent did not eat fruits or vegetables rich in vitamin A, and*
- *82 percent did not eat cruciferous vegetables.*[1]

VITAMINS AND MINERALS: ANTIVIRAL AGENTS

In a study conducted by the U.S. Center for Food Safety and Applied Nutrition, the dietary intakes of eleven nutritional elements for different age groups were assessed. The results?

- *All ages were below established levels for copper.*
- *Six of the eight groups were deficient in magnesium.*
- *Five groups didn't receive enough calcium and zinc.*
- *Teenage groups, on average, were deficient in seven nutrients.*
- *Women failed to meet levels in five nutrients.*
- *Men were below levels in four nutrients.*[2]

As you can see from these studies, most people can use some nutritional supplemental support. Without adequate supplies of certain vitamins and minerals, our natural defense system weakens.

Vitamins: A, B, C, and E

Vitamins are organic compounds your body uses as helpers in various metabolic processes. Each of the thirteen known vitamins has specific health roles. But in terms of military ranking, the top generals in battling viral infections are vitamins A, C, E, and some of the B vitamins.

VITAMIN A

Vitamin A takes on a defensive role by producing special enzymes that are constantly on seek-and-destroy missions against viruses that manage to get inside your body. Ironically, you need vitamin A to live, but you can't produce it on your own. Only plants and specific animal sources like liver contain the ingredients for vitamin A. That's why vitamin A supplements are so important.

Vitamin A enters your body as the vitamin itself and through precursors known as carotenoids. In total, scientists have identified more than 600 carotenoids. The most famous one is beta carotene, the source of the orange color in carrots. Carotenoids

103

got their name because they were first isolated from carrots about a century ago! These compounds are found in colored fruits and vegetables as well as in green plants, legumes, grains, and seeds. They enhance thymus gland function and increase interferon activity.

Vitamin A roles: This versatile vitamin is one of your immune system's truest allies. Among its many functions, vitamin A

- *maintains the health of your mucus membranes and epithelial tissue (plus their secretions), which line the respiratory and digestive tract;*
- *enhances the response of white blood cells and antibodies to viruses;*
- *stimulates the production T cells;*
- *supports proper thymus cell function which, in turn, ensures proper Tcell function; and*
- *is necessary for normal cell division.*[3]

People who are deficient in vitamin A are very prone to viral illnesses. One Long Beach, California, study involving children infected with measles indicated that 50 percent of them were deficient in vitamin A.[4] In a separate study on children, scientists found that infant mortality rates decreased by 50 percent among children who had the measles and were given vitamin A supplements daily.[5]

Children infected with the respiratory syncytial virus (RSV) have also been helped with vitamin A supplements because of an improved immune response to this respiratory tract infection. In short-term use (and with the guidance of your family physician), you can safely give your child 25,000 IUs of vitamin A, without toxic consequences, to eradicate this virus.

In a study among people with AIDS, scientists noted that they often lacked sufficient levels of vitamin A. This shortage may lead to a decreased amount of T helper cells.[6]

Dosages by age: The following table provides the recommended daily value intake of vitamin A by age group.

VITAMINS AND MINERALS: ANTIVIRAL AGENTS

Remember, this is the baseline, based on the minimum amount required for a healthy individual.

Age	Daily Value (in international units)
Infants	
1–3 years	1,875
4–6 years	2,000
7–10 years	2,500
Females, 11 and older	3,500
Males, 11 and older	4,000

Health preventative dosage: 5,000 to 15,000 IUs of vitamin A for adults daily. Or, 25,000 to 50,000 IUs daily of the mixed carotenoid blend.

Viral infection-fighting dosages: 10,000 to 100,000 IUs for infants and children for three to five days maximum. For adults fighting acute viral infections, between 50,000 to 300,000 IUs daily, not to exceed five days.

Caution: Daily dosages of vitamin A should not exceed 5,000 IUs if you are pregnant, unless prescribed by your family physician. High dosages for children must be supervised by a doctor.

Food sources of vitamin A: Once you start taking supplements, don't let them replace food, which contains a lot of valuable nutrients. Here are some excellent food sources containing vitamin A: carrots, sweet potatoes, whole milk, kale, collard greens, parsley, spinach, squash, mangoes, apricots, peaches, liver.

B VITAMINS

Teamwork. That sums up the value of B vitamins. In total, the vitamin B squadron consists of thiamin, riboflavin, niacin, biotin, pantothenic acid, B6, folic acid, and B12. All eight serve

105

as coenzymes to enzymes that dispense energy from proteins, carbohydrates, and fats. All are water-soluble, which means they are directly absorbed into the bloodstream and travel freely throughout the body. Excess amounts are excreted.

The B vitamins are crucial for a properly functioning immune system. Specifically, riboflavin, B6, folic acid, and pantothenic acid are all necessary for the production of antibodies. B6 is particularly important, since the primary food sources for it are grains and vegetables, two areas in which not everyone meets the RDA levels. Having a B6 deficiency can decrease your thymus hormone activity and reduce of the number and activity of lymphocytes and antibodies.[7]

Roles of B vitamins: These vitamins

- *help cells produce energy;*
- *reduce stress;*
- *are involved in many metabolic pathways;*
- *produce antibodies;*
- *help build new cells to deliver oxygen and nutrients; and*
- *are needed by phagocytes to function properly.*

Scientists estimate that up to 35 percent of people infected with HIV are deficient in vitamin B12.[8, 9] These people would benefit from extra vitamin B supplementation.

B Vitamin	Recommended Daily Values (in milligrams and micrograms)
Thiamin	1.5 mg
Riboflavin	1.7 mg
Niacin	20 mg
B6	2 mg
B12	6 mcg
Folic acid	400 mcg
Biotin	300 mcg

VITAMINS AND MINERALS: ANTIVIRAL AGENTS

Recommended dosage: You can obtain a daily supply of the B vitamins by purchasing a quality multivitamin product. (See also the table on page 106.)

Viral infection-fighting dosages: An extra 50 to 100 mg B complex can be helpful for those under stress or needing therapeutic dosages.

Caution: Single B vitamins, when needed, should be prescribed by practitioners of nutritional medicine.

Food sources of B vitamins: Here are some valuable sources of foods containing B vitamins and other essential nutrients: fortified corn flakes, watermelon, sunflower seeds, lean ham, cottage cheese, milk, eggs, shrimp, spinach, broccoli, navy beans, okra, asparagus, and turnip greens.

VITAMIN C

In the world of supplements, vitamin C is the ultimate loyal soldier, ready to sacrifice itself to save the body. Known scientifically as ascorbic acid, vitamin C is probably the most studied vitamin in the world.

Medical experts debate vitamin C's impact on ridding the common cold, but no one doubts this vitamin's antiviral effect and ability to fortify the immune system. Over twenty double-blind studies have demonstrated that vitamin C decreases the duration of the common cold or, at least, reduces the severity of symptoms. Since vitamin C is non-toxic, it would make sense to rely on it as a cold-fighting supplement.

Two-time Nobel laureate Linus Pauling, Ph.D., regarded as the father of the vitamin C movement and author of the best-seller *Vitamin C and the Common Cold*, spent his lifetime conducting studies to support vitamin C's role in enhancing the immune system. He took 12,000 mg of vitamin C in his orange juice every morning and lived to be ninety-three.

Because it is a water-soluble vitamin it is vulnerable to heat, alkalinity, and exposure to air. Supplies of vitamin C can be rapidly depleted within the body during times of extreme physical and emotional stress. Chemical pollutants, including cigarette smoke when exposure is prolonged, can also rob the body of vitamin C. Some medical experts estimate that one cigarette depletes 250 mg of vitamin C. A study in the *Journal of Nutritional Health* stated that physiological, chemical, emotional, and psychological stress significantly increase the urinary excretion of vitamin C.[10–12]

Vitamin C roles: This vitamin

- *serves as an excellent antioxidant, ridding the body of dangerous free radicals;*
- *increases white blood cells in number and accelerates their activity levels;*
- *increases interferon;*
- *stimulates antibody response;*
- *activates thymic hormone secretion;*
- *helps form collagen and strengthens connective tissue; and*
- *metabolizes hormones in the adrenal glands to fight stress.*

Age or Type	Daily Value (in milligrams)
0–6 months	30
6–12 months	35
1–3 years	40
4–10 years	45
11–14 years	50
15 and over	60
Pregnant females	70
Lactating females	95
Smokers	100

Dosages by age and type: The RDA for vitamin C is quite minimal.

Preventation: For optimal health I recommend 500 to 1,500 mg daily of vitamin C.

Viral infection-fighting dosage: Among the aggressive forms of natural medical treatment of hepatitis and AIDS is vitamin C delivered intravenously, according to Robert Cathart, M.D. For the treatment of hepatitis and AIDS, Dr. Cathart recommends intravenous doses of vitamin C between 40 g (40,000 mg) to 100 g (100,000 mg) daily.

Dr. Cathart and other physicians also believe intravenous doses of vitamin C are necessary to cure hepatitis as well. He has shown that these high dosages of vitamin C can substantially improve hepatitis in two to four days and clear jaundice (yellowing of the skin) within six days.[13-16]

For acute infections I recommend taking vitamin C up to bowel tolerance. Take higher doses of vitamin C until diarrhea begins, then cut back to a dosage that does not cause this symptom. This range differs for everybody. The dosages should be divided in amounts of 1,000 mg every two to three hours. For severe infections like Hepatitis, intravenous vitamin C is recommended, to be administered by a physician. For individuals sensitive to vitamin C (especially people with citrus and acid food sensitivity) I recommend use of a non-acidic form of vitamin C called "Ester C."

Caution: How much vitamin C is too much? The method of determining the proper dose for the treatment of disease, by increasing gradually to bowel tolerance, will determine this. Although it is hard to take too much vitamin C, levels 30 times or higher than the Daily Value can lead to cramps, diarrhea, and, possibly, kidney stone formation.

Food sources of vitamin C: Good sources include Acerola cherries, chili peppers, kale, parsley, collard greens, broccoli, oranges, cantaloupes, strawberries, papayas, and mangoes.

NATURE'S VIRUS KILLERS

VITAMIN E

Unquestionably, vitamin E is the most important fat-soluble antioxidant. Just as its cousin vitamin C is effective against to the common cold, vitamin E has been hailed for its tremendous benefits in maintaining the cardiovascular system. Inside cell membranes, it exerts antioxidant effects against pollutants.

But among its many other duties, vitamin E also enhances and protects the immune system. It delivers protection for the thymus gland and white blood cells, and helps support and protect the immune system during chronic viral illnesses.

Vitamin E roles: This vitamin

- *acts as a super antioxidant;*
- *is required for phagocyte and antibody activity;*
- *improves the immune system by protecting red and white blood cells;*
- *aids in cellular respiration;*
- *protects lungs from pollutants;*
- *protects lipids; and*
- *helps heal scar tissue.*[17]

Dosages by age and type: The RDA for vitamin E is quite minimal.

Age or Type	Daily Value (in international units)
0–1 year	
1–10 years	4.5–6.0
Males, 11 and older	9.0–10.5
Females, 11 and older	15.0
Pregnant females	12.0
Lactating females	15.0
	18.0

Prevention dosage: I recommend taking 400 to 800 IU daily. Make sure to use a natural source of vitamin E, known as d-alpha tocopherol. Synthetic sources are not as effective.

Caution: If you are on a blood-thinning medication like coumadin, check with your physician first before using.

Food sources of vitamin E: You can find plenty of this vitamin in polyunsaturated plant oils, nuts, whole grains, vegetable oils, and green leafy vegetables.

Minerals: Selenium, Zinc, and Coenzyme Q10

Minerals are inorganic elements that always keep their chemical identities. Once minerals enter your body, they stay there until excreted. They cannot be converted into energy as protein or carbohydrates can. Once selenium, always selenium.

Major minerals such as calcium, phosphorus, and magnesium are found in large quantities in your body. Trace minerals, (such as iron, selenium, and zinc) as their name implies, occur in small amounts.

SELENIUM

Small but mighty, that's the motto for this trace mineral. It acts as an antioxidant and is very necessary to prevent viral infections and enhance immune function. A deficiency of selenium is an invitation to viruses to replicate and thrive.

A 1994 study by Kiremidjian-Scumacher et al., examined individuals with normal levels of selenium in their blood. Scientists then had this group take 200 micrograms of selenium supplements daily. This added amount of selenium resulted in an astounding 118-percent increase in the ability of lymphocytes to kill tumor cells and an 82-percent increase in natural killer cells to destroy cancer cells and various pathogens.[18]

Selenium is like a foot soldier belonging to the antioxidant defense system of the body.

Selenium roles: This mineral

- *supports white blood cell function;*
- *acts as an antioxidant; and*
- *supports thymus function.*

Dosages by age and type:

Age or Type	Daily Value (in micrograms)
0–6 months	10
6–12 months	15
1–6 years	20
7–10 years	30
Males, 11–14	40
Males, 15–18	50
Males, 19 and older	70
Females, 11–14	45
Females, 15–18	50
Females, 19 and older	55
Pregnant females	65
Lactating females	75

Preventation dosage: I recommend adults take up to 200 micrograms of selenium daily. For children, the amount is 1.5 micrograms for every pound they weigh.

Viral infection-fighting dosages: Take 400 micrograms during a viral infection and 200 micrograms as a preventative dosage.

Caution: There is no need to take high dosages of trace minerals such as selenium. Higher than recommended dosages can result in toxic symptoms. Fortunately, cases of severe selenium toxicity are rare in the United States.

Food sources of selenium: You'll find rich amounts of selenium in clams, crabs, lobsters, oysters, whole grains, wheat germs, Brazil nuts, oats, and bran.

VITAMINS AND MINERALS: ANTIVIRAL AGENTS

ZINC

This mineral really gets around. Essentially, every cell in your body contains zinc, with the highest concentrations in bone, the eyes, and the prostate gland. Think of zinc as the body's workhorse. It is involved in more than 300 enzymatic reactions.

Zinc roles: This mineral

- *keeps the thymus gland functioning properly;*
- *keeps white blood cells functioning properly;*
- *fights cold viruses;*
- *maintains healthy skin;*
- *assists platelets in blood clotting; and*
- *protects the body from heavy metal poisoning.*

People who exercise often, drink large amounts of alcohol, are under a lot of stress, or vegetarians are prime targets for zinc deficiency. Why? Zinc levels are easily lost through sweat and urine. Low levels of zinc can lead to decreased T lymphocytes, lower thymic hormone, and decreased white blood cell function. Fortunately, zinc supplementation can reverse these effects.[19]

Dosages by age and type:

Age or Type	Daily Value (in milligrams)
Infants under 1 year	5
1–10 years	10
Males, 11 and older	15
Females, 11 and older	12
Pregnant females	15
Lactating females	19

Prevention dosage: Adults should take 15 to 30 mg daily as a prevention against disease.

NATURE'S VIRUS KILLERS

Viral infection-fighting dosages: Take 50 mg daily.

Caution: Taking excessively high amounts of zinc—2 grams or more—may lead to diarrhea, vomiting, fever, and exhaustion.

Food sources of zinc: Good sources include oysters, shellfish, fish, red meat, whole grains, legumes, nuts, and seeds.

COENZYME Q10

Coenzyme Q10 is a vitamin-like substance with a science-fiction-sounding name. Nicknamed CoQ10, it acts as a powerful antioxidant and is necessary for energy production within cells. Its main job is to convert food into energy.

Coenzyme Q10 roles: This substance

- *increases antibody production;*
- *improves macrophage activity;*
- *boosts energy production within cells;*
- *serves as an antioxidant;*
- *strengthens heart muscles; and*
- *transforms food you eat into energy for your body.*[20]

Dosage by age: There is no Recommended Daily Value established for coenzyme Q10. However, I advise adults to take 30 to 120 mg of coenzyme Q10 daily as a health promoting dosage.

Viral infection-fighting dosage: 100 to 300 mg daily.

Caution: This is generally regarded as a safe and non-toxic nutrient.

Food sources of coenzyme Q10: Found in oily fish, organ meats, whole grains, and peanuts.

Chapter 8
HOMEOPATHY: PLACEBO OR POTENT VIRUS DESTROYER?

~~~~~~

How does homeopathy work?
What homeopathic medicines work best against viruses?
Who was Dr. Samuel Hahnemann?
What guidelines should one follow?

O f all the different types of natural medicines, homeopathy is unquestionably the most controversial. Homeopathy is a unique system of medicine that uses remedies made from vegetable, mineral, animal, and other sources to treat illness and prevent disease. Most of these remedies are so highly diluted that none of the original material is left in the medicine. The philosophy behind using ultra-diluted substances is to stimulate the immune response in the treatment and prevention of disease.

Many scientists now believe that each homeopathic remedy has its own "fingerprint" on the electromagnetic spectrum. In other words, homeopathic remedies work on a vibrational level. Like acupuncture in some ways, each remedy has a different frequency and thus action, as with the different actions of various acupuncture points.

Homeopathy is not a new system of medicine. In fact, Hindu literature describes the homeopathic effect in tenth-century B.C. In 400 B.C. Greece, Hippocrates wrote about the principles of homeopathy, stating, "Through the like, disease is produced and through the application of the like, it is cured."

NATURE'S VIRUS KILLERS

Homeopathy gained widespread acceptance in the early 1800s through the leadership of German medical doctor and chemist Samuel Hahnemann. Dr. Hahnemann was passionate about developing a safer, more effective system of medicine for his patients. He abandoned his conventional medical practice because he believed the medical therapies of his time were too barbaric. He did not believe in bloodletting or using high doses of mercury or arsenic on his patients, because of the dangerous consequences.

A scholar as well as a translator of books from different languages, Dr. Hahnemann came upon the writings of homeopathy, which piqued his curiosity. Historical references indicate that Dr. Hahnemann's interest arose after reading a book that stated that cinchona bark would cure malaria because of its bitter taste. Not satisfied with this explanation, Dr. Hahnemann tried an experiment on himself. After taking successive doses of cinchona bark, he developed symptoms of sweating, chills, fatigue, and weakness. These are the same symptoms as malaria. This experiment led him to the realization that "like cures like."

The word homeopathy comes from the Greek root words *homoios,* which means similar, and *pathos,* which means suffering or disease. This relates to the fundamental law of homeopathy—"like cures like." This means a substance that can cause particular symptoms in healthy people can stimulate healing in those who are ill with similar symptoms. Let me illustrate using the herb belladonna (which is toxic and should not be ingested). When taken by a healthy person, belladonna causes symptoms of fever, flushed face, and dilated pupils. However, the homeopathic preparation of belladonna (ultra-diluted and specially shaken) is very helpful for a person who is ill and exhibits these same symptoms. The diluted belladonna helps stimulate the immune system to fight off the infections.

Not convinced? Okay, let's take another example using the homeopathic apis, a preparation of bee venom. The common symptoms of a bee sting are stinging, burning, redness, and swelling. These are the same symptoms that can be relieved by the homeopathic apis. In fact, apis works on these symptoms when also caused by arthritis or a urinary tract infection. If the symptoms match those of the homeopathic, a cure can occur as the body's healing mechanisms are activated by the law of similars.

Homeopathy is used as a primary form of medicine all over the world. In India, there are more than 120 homeopathic medical schools, thousands of homeopathic practitioners, and millions of people who use homeopathy every year. In Europe more than half of all doctors prescribe homeopathic medicines or refer to practitioners who use homeopathy. Even members of the royal family demand that their medical treatment include homeopathy! London is home to a prestigious homeopathic hospital and research institute.

As you can see, millions of people throughout the world have experienced the benefits of homeopathy. Its long history has actually led to the development of the pharmaceutical medications used today. In the past decade homeopathy has begun to gain acceptance in mainstream medicine. Physicians, and their patients who are tired and discouraged by prescriptions with toxic side effects, are turning to homeopathy.

Homeopathy offers non-toxic, effective medicine that has the backing of modern scientific research to prove its clinical benefits. As a physician trained in both conventional and natural medicine, I rate homeopathy as one of my most trusted forms of treatment for all types of health conditions. Specifically for viral infections, homeopathy seems almost miraculous at times, as you will notice in some of my case studies provided later in this chapter.

LESS IS STRONGER

Dr. Hahnemann and other medical practitioners have found that homeopathy becomes more effective and powerful when prepared by a special process of dilution and sucussion (shaking or pounding of the medicines). This process is referred to as potentization and indicates the strength of a homeopathic. Special laboratory equipment is used in homeopathic pharmacies and research centers to produce homeopathic remedies with this special technique.

WORKING WITH THE BODY

Homeopathy is unique in that it works with the healing systems of the body. For viral infections, the correct homeopathic remedy stimulates the immune system to overcome the invading pathogen. This is a better remedy than antibiotics, which directly kill bacteria (but are powerless against viruses) but do nothing to harness the power of the immune system.

As we go into depth later in this chapter, you will learn that homeopathic medicines are prescribed not only for a disease itself (such as the flu or measles) but also for symptoms that are expressed by the person. As I stated in my book, *The Natural Physician*, there are four reasons why I believe homeopathy is gaining popularity:

- *Homeopathy is highly effective for chronic and acute diseases, including epidemics. It works to strengthen the immune system and can treat viruses and other conditions for which conventional medicine has no effective treatment.*
- *It is cost effective. Compared to pharmaceutical medications, homeopathic remedies are quite inexpensive.*
- *It is a preventative medicine. One does not have to have a disease to be treated with homeopathy. It can be used to optimize health.*
- *It can be used to treat the whole person. Homeopathy takes into account all the factors of a person's health—the mental, emotional, and physical.*[1]

PRESCRIBING HOMEOPATHY

There are two basic ways I recommend my patients or the public use homeopathy:

Combination remedies. This refers to homeopathic formulas that contain two or more homeopathic remedies. If the one a person needs is in the formula, then it will be helpful. If the homeopathic remedy a person needs is not one of the ingredients, then usually nothing will happen. Combination remedies are available in most health food stores or pharmacies. They are prepared for certain conditions, including colds, flu, premenstrual syndrome, menopause, headaches, and others.

Single remedies. This is the system used by most homeopathic practitioners—the one remedy that matches up best to the patient's symptoms is prescribed. In general, this system is more effective than combination remedies, but requires a knowledgeable practitioner to pick the correct homeopathic.

HOW TO USE HOMEOPATHICS

Homeopathic remedies are generally available in pellet, tablet, liquid, or cream form. They are best taken at least ten minutes after eating or drinking—not before or after. They are also best taken when away from strong smelling odors such as eucalyptus.

For acute conditions, homeopathic remedies are often taken every fifteen minutes or two hours, depending on the severity of the condition. For chronic conditions, homeopathics are usually taken one to two times daily, or less frequently, depending on the strength of the remedy prescribed.

UNDERSTANDING DIFFERENT STRENGTHS OF REMEDIES

Potency refers to the strength of the remedy. The number behind the name of the homeopathic indicates the dilution and strength of the medicine. The higher the number, the stronger the action of the remedy. For example, 30C is stronger than 15C.

The two common scales of homeopathy available to the public are

- *"X," indicates the lowest potencies used. X stands for a 1 in 9 dilution. 1X is equal to 1 part of the original substance diluted in 9 parts solvent.*
- *"C," is more dilute and stronger than the X potencies. The first dilution, that is, 1C, is equal to 1 part of the original substance in 99 parts of solvent.*

Common homeopathic remedies used for acute viral diseases

Let's say you're trying to shake a bad cold or sore throat, or you can't seem to clear a nagging ear or kidney infection. Newcomers should certainly consult a natural health-care practitioner first, but what follows are eight homeopathic remedies that are commonly used to treat various viral infections. Symptoms and conditions treated are listed for each.

Aconite (Aconitum napellus)—monkshood
- *Symptoms come on very quickly and intensely, and almost always at the beginning of an infection.*
- *Person exhibits panic, restlessness, and fear of death with the infection or illness.*
- *One cheek may be red and the other cheek pale.*
- *Great thirst for cold drinks.*

Common infectious conditions: cold, flu, sore throat, ear infection, bladder infection, measles.

Apis (Apis mellifica)—honey bee
- *Stinging, burning, redness, and swelling are the key physical symptoms.*
- *Feels better with cool applications and worse with warm applications.*
- *Thirstless.*

Common infectious conditions: sore throat, bladder infection, kidney infection, shingles, herpes, pneumonia, chicken pox.

Arsenicum (Arsenicum album)—arsenic trioxide
- *Tremendous anxiety, with restlessness.*
- *Chilly and burning pains that are better with warmth.*
- *Fever from midnight to early in the morning.*

Common infectious conditions: bronchitis, bladder infection, hepatitis, herpes, cold, flu, kidney infection, pneumonia, shingles, and upper respiratory infection.

120

HOMEOPATHY: PLACEBO OR POTENT VIRUS DESTROYER?

Belladonna
- *High fever, flushed face, dilated pupils, and throbbing pain.*
- *Low thirst.*
- *Cold hands and feet but hot face.*

Common infectious conditions: fever, bladder infections, kidney infections, ear infections, tonsillitis, sore throats.

Ferrum phos (Ferrum phophoricum)—phosphate of iron
- *Fever, flushed face, and fatigue.*
- *Person may have a fever but not act sick.*

Common infectious conditions: cold, flu, ear infection.

Gelsemium (Gelsemium sempervirens)—yellow jasmine
- *Weakness, fatigue, and aching of the muscles.*
- *Chills.*
- *Thirstless.*

Common infectious conditions: chronic fatigue, mononucleosis, Epstein-Barr virus, flu.

Mercury (Mercurius vivus)—quicksilver
- *Heavy perspiration, alternating with chills.*
- *Intolerant to hot and cold temperatures.*
- *Foul breath and metallic taste in mouth.*
- *Increased salivation and dirty coating on tongue.*

Common infectious conditions: flu, ear infection, cold, upper respiratory infection, bladder infection.

Pulsatilla (Pulsatilla pratensis)—windflower
- *Fever with low thirst.*
- *Feels better with company and comfort.*
- *Yellow/green mucous discharge.*

Common infectious conditions: ear infection, sore throat, bronchitis.[2]

Obviously, in all these cases listed, the exact choice of the homeopathic remedy depends on the individual person and the specific symptoms that he or she exhibits.

NATURE'S VIRUS KILLERS

Now let me share with you some success stories involving my patients who used homeopathy.

CASE STUDY 1

Melissa, fourteen, was struck by a flu-like illness that was compounded by weeks of excruciating headaches. Conventional doctors performed comprehensive exams, including an MRI that ruled out a brain infection or brain hemorrhage. Blood work showed signs of a viral infection. Unable to go to school for two months because of debilitating headaches, Melissa came to see me with her mother. They were frustrated. Antibiotics, migraine prescriptions, and other therapies weren't working.

It was evident to me that a viral infection had penetrated Melissa's immune system and was causing the headaches. My recommendation was the homeopathic medicine Scutellaria 30C, to be taken twice daily for one week. The indications for Scutellaria include weakness, headaches, or never getting well since the onset of the flu or viral illness. Melissa's mother called back in one week to joyously explain that Melissa's headaches were gone after five days of taking Scutellaria. The Scutellaria invoked an immune response against the viral infection. Melissa went on to recover nicely after the remedy.

CASE STUDY 2

A retired judge sought my help with what was diagnosed by his medical doctor as a viral intestinal infection. After vacationing in Mexico, he suffered from severe fatigue, nausea, abdominal cramps, chills, and irritability. Antibiotics didn't work. I prescribed the homeopathic Nux Vomica. This medicine is indicated for intestinal cramps that accompany a flu or viral infection. Two days later, his fatigue, chills, and digestive symptoms were gone.

CASE STUDY 3

When I first met Tyler, this three-year-old was crying from the pain of a severe ear infection. He had a high fever of 105 degrees

HOMEOPATHY: PLACEBO OR POTENT VIRUS DESTROYER?

Fahrenheit. His face was flushed; he tugged at his right ear; and his pupils were slightly dilated. Based on Tyler's symptoms, I immediately prescribed the homeopathic Belladonna. Within ten minutes, Tyler fell asleep. In twenty minutes, his temperature dropped to 100 degrees. By the next morning, Tyler was up and playing as if nothing had happened. Belladonna is one of the excellent homeopathic medicines for acute infections (viral or bacterial) where there is fever, flushed face, and an intensity of symptoms.

Chapter 9

COMPLEMENTARY THERAPIES: ACUPUNCTURE, HYDROTHERAPY, AND THE MIND-BODY CONNECTION

~~~~~~

What is acupuncture?
How does hydrotherapy fight viruses?
How does stress affect my immune system?
What is mental imagery?

Acupuncture

Time is acupuncture's ally. Even though western medicine regards it as a "new alternative" therapy, acupuncture has been a well-respected form of treatment for nearly 5,000 years in Eastern cultures.

By the simplest of definitions, acupuncture is the insertion of very fine needles into specific spots on the skin, with the goal of affecting physiological functioning of the body.

The first record of acupuncture dates back 4,700 years, when it was described in the *Huang Di Nei Jing (Yellow Emperor's Classic of Internal Medicine)*, considered to be the world's oldest medical textbook. In this book, theories of acupuncture are outlined by Shen Nung, the father of Chinese medicine. He wrote about circulation, the heart, and pulse centuries ahead of European medical writings.

Shen Nung believed that inside the body is an energy force called *qi* (pronounced "chee") that consists of all essential life activities: physical, mental, emotional, and spiritual. *Qi* flows through the body along special pathways, known as meridians or channels, with designated acupuncture points located throughout the body. When *qi* is flowing properly through the meridians, a person can harmonize the healing abilities of his or her body.

According to Chinese medical theory, illness arises when the flow of *qi* is inadequate, interrupted, or out of balance.

Acupuncture, as well as acupressure (in which specific body points are massaged or pressed on), help re-establish optimal *qi* flow. There are well over 365 acupuncture points along fourteen main meridians in the body. When an acupuncture needle, or acupressure, is applied to one of these points, any blockage of *qi* is cleared, so that the energy flow is fully restored.

Acupuncture or acupressure can be used for both acute viral illnesses and chronic conditions. Points are selected based on a person's symptoms, in order to expel the invading pathogen. However, acupuncture and acupressure represent only a small part of Chinese medicine. Chinese herbal therapy, *qi gong*, diet, and other therapeutic treatments are very important components as well.

Today, holistic health practitioners and an increasing number of conventional physicians incorporate acupuncture and Oriental medicine in their practices to treat viral conditions and a host of other health problems. The World Health Organization lists more than forty health conditions that benefit from the use of acupuncture. In 1997, the National Institutes of Health conducted studies and concluded that acupuncture is effective for a number of conditions, including lower-back pain, tennis elbow, post-surgery nausea, chemotherapy nausea, and dental surgery pain.[1]

Among the most common conditions treated successfully with acupuncture and acupressure are headaches, arthritis, allergies, muscle spasms, anxiety, depression, and drug and alcohol addictions.[2]

So, how does acupuncture work? Despite its long history, medical experts are still grappling for explanations. However, here are some of the prevailing theories:

- *Acupuncture elevates levels of white blood cells, specific hormones, prostaglandins, gamma globulins, antibodies, and opsonins.*
- *Acupuncture constricts and dilates blood vessels, promoting the body's release of vasodilaters (known as histamines).*
- *Acupuncture activates the secretions of endorphins (the body's "feel-good" hormones), specifically enkaphalins.*
- *Acupuncture elevates the levels of neurotransmitters, specifically serotonin and noradrenaline.[3]*

SPECIFIC ACUPUNCTURE POINTS

There are many acupuncture points that benefit the immune system. The selection is always individualized, based on the diagnosis and examination of a trained practitioner.

Keeping this in mind, here are some common points known to enhance immune function:

Governing vessel 14: This point, nicknamed the "great hammer," is located in the space between the seventh cervical vertebrae of the neck and the first thoracic vertebrae. It is at the bottom of neck where you can feel these vertebrae stick out when you bend your neck forward. Many practitioners state that this point stimulates white blood cell activity.

Gall bladder 39: Located three inches above the outside ankle bone between the bone and tendon in the area, this point is believed to support bone-marrow production for immune cells.

Large intestine 4: This is a popular point used to address many health conditions. It is located in the mound of flesh between the thumb and index finger when they are pulled together side by side. This point is particularly effective for infections that result in high fevers and sweating. By pushing on this point, one can help reduce a fever and stimulate the immune system.

127

ACUPUNCTURE CASE HISTORY

George, an engineer, was recently diagnosed with hepatitis C. Lab tests confirmed that his liver enzymes were elevated, signifying liver damage. He appeared very tired and complained of having a lot of gas and bloating. These were due to decreased liver function.

He came to me for alternative therapies to deal with this serious condition. Taking a comprehensive approach, I suggested dietary changes as well as the introduction of two key liver-supporting herbs: milk thistle and bupleurum. I also arranged for George to receive regular acupuncture treatments. After three treatments, George noticed that his energy improved. After seven treatments, he expressed amazement over his increased energy level and improved digestion.

I explained to George that acupuncture is a standard treatment for hepatitis in China. It is not known exactly how, but acupuncture improves immune function. Stimulation of the acupuncture needles in strategic points awakens the immune system, in part from certain messages from the nervous system and brain. George's liver enzyme counts continue to decrease as he continues his acupuncture treatments.

HYDROTHERAPY

Hydrotherapy is a natural treatment using water internally and externally to promote wellness and healing, which dates back to the days of ancient Greece. In modern times, an Austrian priest named Vincent Priessnitz (1799–1852) is credited with developing naturopathic hydrotherapy.

He discovered it by observing how injured animals on his farm would instinctively soak their injuries in cold water. Then, at age seventeen, he broke two ribs, and a local doctor told him that he could not help him. So Priessnitz applied hydrotherapy techniques to his chest and quickly recovered from his injuries. During his lifetime, he helped thousands with hydrotherapy treatments and diet tips.

The promotion of hydrotherapy to North America was credited to Dr. Benedict Lust (1872–1945), a German immigrant known as the "Father of Naturopathy."

Today, more than ever, people are turning to hydrotherapy as a natural method of healing.

In hydrotherapy, various water forms are used: hot, cold, steam, and ice. Different techniques are applied: whirlpools, wraps, towels, poultices, colonic irrigations, and fomentations. The goal is to apply different water temperatures in various methods to relieve a host of conditions. Among them are nasal congestion, insomnia, colds, the flu, headaches, and stress.

How does it work? Basically the idea behind hydrotherapy is to stimulate white blood cells in your body enough so that they will battle invading viruses. The effective technique of hot and cold water optimizes the circulation of blood and lymph. Short-term use of heat hydrotherapy stimulates and dilates the blood vessels. This action increases oxygenation and the excretion of tissue waste products. Short-term use of cold hydrotherapy elevates white blood cells, enhances tissue oxygenation, and expels waste.

Generally, hydrotherapy can provide these benefits:

- *Detoxify by helping to transport and eliminate toxins from the body through the lymph system, circulatory system, liver, kidneys, digestive tract, and skin.*
- *Relieve stress.*
- *Improve blood circulation to affected areas.*
- *Replenish minerals and nutrients by opening pores and allowing concentrated nutrients (such as those in seaweed baths) to be absorbed into the body.*

Now, let's look at specific ways hydrotherapy can provide benefits. You can make a sinus headache vanish, for example, by placing both feet in a container of warm water while placing an ice pack around the neck. Two things are happening: the warm water is dilating the blood vessels in the feet, which increases blood flow there and moves the congested blood away from the head. At the same time, the ice pack is constricting the blood vessels in the neck and head area to relieve congestion.

To evoke an immune-system response by enhancing a fever reaction, you can use the proper application of hot and cold hydrotherapy techniques. Remember, a fever stimulates your immune system to fight viral invaders and toxins.

For general tonification such as cancer treatments, overall body hydrotherapy can help. Cancer is regarded as the systemic breakdown of the immune system. Hydrotherapy, conversely, is the stimulator of the immune system.

Please refer to Appendix I, p. 167, for detailed instructions on constitutional hydrotherapy and foot hydrotherapy.

HYDROTHERAPY CASE STUDY

Jerry, a forty-five-year-old teacher, came to my clinic for a bad cough that had been uncontrollable for three days. An examination and chest X ray revealed that Jerry had viral pneumonia. I prescribed constitutional hydrotherapy as one of Jerry's primary treatment plans. Every day, Jerry underwent hydrotherapy treatments; he noticed that his symptoms began subsiding. The hydrotherapy helped to loosen up and expel mucus from his lungs. The alternation of the hot and cold compresses on his chest area helped to reduce the pain and inflammation. It also enlisted the aid of his army of immune cells to fight off the infection.

MIND-BODY CONNECTION

The best partnership you will ever have exists between your mind and your body. One of the most underrated tools in immune system enhancement and for general health is the healing power of the mind.

Visualization and mental imagery are two techniques that use the power of positive thoughts to relieve pain, control illness, and attain goals. At the root of these approaches is the relaxation response. This is important to counter the harmful effects of stress. After all, one cannot be in both a state of stress and a state of relaxation.

130

Visualization is the technique that allows you to picture a scene in your mind. It could be seeing yourself crossing the finish line after a fifty-mile bike race or completing a complicated project at work—ahead of schedule. What you're doing is rehearsing success rather than failure. This feel-good attitude strengthens the endorphins and other hormones that keep your immune system healthy.

Imagery is a more detailed technique that not only involves you picturing a scene in your mind, but also tapping into your other senses: taste, smell, sound, and touch. The goal behind imagery is being able to put yourself in another place for a period of time, a place that allows you to relax. After facing a stress-filled day of deadlines and obligations, spend a few minutes and imagine yourself sitting on the banks of a peaceful creek on a cool day with a mild breeze, the smell of wildflowers and the sounds of birds chirping all around you. By locking into this image (or another favorite), you are distracting yourself from stressful situations and helping your body to heal and fortify itself.

The power of controlled thought can affect your body's heart rate, blood pressure, temperature, muscle relaxation, immune system, oxygen consumption, and gastrointestinal activity. More and more, scientific studies are noting the health link between one's physical and mental states.

Cancer and immune-enhancement clinics around the world are using the science of psychoneuroimmunology (based on the relationship of the mind's connection to the nervous system and its connection to the immune system) to enhance the body's immunity. Many physicians are recommending that patients envision themselves getting healthier by picturing fighter cells attacking cancer cells or gobbling up invading viruses and pathogens.

How you handle everyday stress can also affect your chances of developing common medical conditions such as colds. Studies have documented that stress can weaken your resistance to viral infections. In fact, constant worry or anxiety can elevate your susceptibility to catching a cold by up to 90 percent! Visualization and imagery can help you keep stress from dictating your thoughts and harming your health.

NATURE'S VIRUS KILLERS

Whether you are practicing visualization or imagery, follow these guidelines for success:

- *Wear loose-fitting, comfortable clothes.*
- *Select a quiet place where you won't be interrupted for five to ten minutes (away from telephones, televisions, etc.).*
- *Sit in a recliner or comfortable chair.*
- *Inhale slowly, drawing air through your nose. Keep your mouth closed. Breathe deeply, all the way down into your belly.*
- *Before slowly exhaling, count to five.*
- *As you exhale through your nose, let your stomach and chest muscles relax. Your shoulders should drop as well.*
- *Continue this inhale-exhale cycle for about five to ten minutes while you practice visualization or imagery. (thinking of an image that is pleasurable and relaxing for you).*
- *Set aside five to ten minutes each day to practice mental imagery.*

Chapter 10
COMMON VIRAL INFECTIONS AND NATURAL SOLUTIONS

~~~~~~

What are the most common viral infections?
How can I treat bronchitis naturally?
What herbs treat chicken pox?
What are the best vitamins for shingles?

Congratulations! You're ready to take more control of your health! In the previous chapters, I've shared with you how viruses affect your immune system and how integrating healthy habits with natural medicine and techniques can keep most, if not all, of these nasty invaders at bay.

This final chapter puts all the pieces together and provides specific ways to treat the most common viral infections facing you and your family today.

Just a few reminders before you plunge ahead. Specific dosages and frequency of use are based on the average adult weighing 150 pounds. Use that as your benchmark. Don't hesitate to consult your naturopathic physician or other holistic health-care practitioner for a specific dosage that meets your special needs. Treatment by a natural-medicine practitioner is advised whenever possible for optimal results.

Accessibility is a big plus in my solution plan. Most of these herbal medicines, vitamins, minerals, homeopathic remedies, and other natural treatments are readily available at your local health-food store or pharmacy (or even your supermarket, in some cases). They are also safer and, often times, less expensive than conventional prescriptive medications.

133

NATURE'S VIRUS KILLERS

As a bonus, the virus cocktail (see Chapter 3) improves your immune system for *all* of these conditions.

You play the most pivotal role in all of these treatments. Stop waiting and hoping for the viral infections to disappear on their own. Here is the ammunition you need to enhance your immune system with natural treatments that will contain or eradicate viral invaders.

Here are the thirteen viral conditions that top my Body Enemy List:

- *Bronchitis*
- *Chicken pox*
- *Common cold*
- *Hepatitis*
- *HIV/AIDS*
- *Measles*
- *Mononucleosis (Epstein-Barr)*
- *Meningitis*
- *Mumps*
- *Pneumonia*
- *Shingles*
- *Sore throat (pharyngitis)*
- *Warts*

Bronchitis

What it is: Bronchitis refers to an infection and inflammation of the passageway leading to the lungs known as the bronchi. Common symptoms include fever, fatigue, and coughing. The cough can be dry or produce mucus. This condition is commonly caused by viral and bacterial infections.

Caution: Although bronchitis responds well to natural treatments, do not confuse it with bronchiolitis. This condition is caused by a specific viral infection (known as RSV) in the lower respiratory tract of infants and young children. It usually develops after a few days of cold symptoms. Symptoms can include wheezing and respiratory distress. It requires immediate medical attention and possible hospitalization to prevent respiratory failure. Bronchiolitis requires medical supervision, including the use of natural therapies.

TREATMENT PLANS FOR BRONCHITIS:

Herbal
- Echinacea or echinacea/goldenseal: 60 drops or 500 mg every three hours.
- Olive leaf extract: 500 mg every three hours.
- Astragalus: 60 drops or 500 mg every three hours.
- Mullein: 30 drops every three hours to soothe lung pain.
- Cherry bark extract: 500 mg or 30 drops every three hours to reduce cough.

Vitamins and Minerals
- Vitamin C: 1000 mg every three hours (cut back if diarrhea occurs).
- Vitamin A: 100,000 IUs daily for three days and then reduce to 50,000 IU daily.
- Zinc: 50 mg daily.

135

NATURE'S VIRUS KILLERS

Nutrition

- Eat chicken soup, broths, ginger, garlic, and onions. Drink at least 8 ounces of water a day. Avoid sugary foods.

Homeopathy (for specific symptoms)

- Phosphorous: burning in lungs, feeling better with cold drinks.
- Antimonium tart: lots of mucus in lungs, rattling of mucus in chest.
- Arsenicum: chills, restlessness, shortness of breath, fatigue.
- Sulphur: burning in lungs, feeling hot and sweaty, last stage of pneumonia.
- Bryonia: sharp sticking pains in chest, feeling chilly.

Other Natural Treatments

- Acupuncture and Chinese herbal therapy from a practitioner.
- Constitutional hydrotherapy.

Chicken Pox

What it is: This acute, highly contagious disease is caused by the Varicella-zoster virus. Epidemics of chicken pox among children usually occur in winter and early spring. This condition is easily spread through respiratory droplets released when talking, sneezing, and coughing. Symptoms of fatigue, fever, muscle aches, and a mild headache usually surface in a person about fifteen days after being exposed to the virus. At that point, an itchy rash of red dots appears (usually starting on the face and torso and then spreading to the rest of the body). Blisters form and develop into scabs that flake off within a week or two.

Caution: Chicken pox is generally a much more severe and painful infection for adults than children. Complications are rare unless the infected person is pregnant. The virus can cause problems for the fetus. Fortunately, most people develop chicken pox during childhood, and it is very rare to be re-infected later in life.

TREATMENT PLANS FOR CHICKEN POX:

Note: Dosages are targeted for children, since they get chicken pox more than adults.

Herbal
- Echinacea/goldenseal: 20 to 30 drops or 500 mg every three hours.
- Olive leaf extract: 250 to 500 mg every three hours. Both herbs help prevent infected lesions.

Herbal topical application—Option 1: Oat bath. Add a cup of oatmeal powder (such as Aveno) to a warm bath. Soak in the tub for at least five minutes. Do not rinse off after stepping out of the tub. Pat dry. Leave a film of oats (*Avena sativa*), which contain anti-itch properties, on the body.

137

Herbal topical application—Option 2: Sock of oatmeal. Fill a sock or porous bag with oatmeal, tie it under the faucet, and run water over it during the bath. Soak in the tub for at least five minutes. Add peppermint (*Mentha piperita*) essential oil to the bath for additional anti-itch and antiseptic benefits.

Vitamins and Minerals
- Vitamin C: 250 to 500 mg every three hours for immune system support and skin healing.
- Vitamin A: 25,000 IUs daily until skin has healed over.

Nutrition
- Eat chicken soup, broths, ginger, garlic, and onions. Drink at least 8 ounces of water a day. Avoid sugary foods.

Homeopathy (for specific symptoms)
- Variolinum: speeds up the course of the disease and is helpful in preventing a painful outbreak. Take as soon as possible.
- Rhus toxicodendron: helpful for the intense itching and restlessness. Take twice daily until there is relief of symptoms.
- Sulphur: Use if Rhus toxicodendron does not provide relief, especially if there is burning pain.

Common Cold

What it is: This condition is caused by a variety of viruses that infect the upper respiratory system. About 30 to 50 percent of all colds are caused by the rhinovirus (which has over one hundred different varieties). Symptoms usually begin with throat or nasal discomfort, followed by sneezing, runny nose, headache, and fatigue. Left untreated, symptoms usually resolve in four to ten days when there are no complications such as sinusitis or ear infections. When natural treatments are begun during the first stage of cold symptoms, they can disappear quickly—sometimes within one to four hours! You can reduce the length and severity of a cold with natural therapies during any stage.

Caution: Conventional treatments (over-the-counter medications) help against symptoms, but do not reduce the length of a cold. In fact, many over-the-counter pharmaceutical decongestants have been shown to actually increase the duration of a cold by providing a breeding ground for the infecting virus!

TREATMENT PLANS FOR COMMON COLDS:

Herbal
- Echinacea: 60 drops or 500 mg every two to three hours.
- Olive leaf extract: 500 mg every two to three hours.
- Astragalus: 60 drops or 500 mg every two to three hours.
- Lomatium: 30 to 60 drops or 500 mg every two to three hours.
- Elderberry: 60 drops or 500 mg every two to three hours.
- Ginger tea: sip cups throughout the day.

Note: Use one or a combination of these herbs as found in formulas.

NATURE'S VIRUS KILLERS

Vitamins and Minerals
- Vitamin C: 1,000 mg every three hours (cut back if diarrhea occurs).
- Zinc lozenge: 15 mg lozenge, three to four times daily
Note: Regular supplementation with a multivitamin has been shown to reduce the frequency of colds, especially in the elderly.

Nutrition
- Eat chicken soup, broths, and drink at least 8 ounce of water daily. Eat plenty of ginger, garlic, and onions, as these foods give immune-system support.

Homeopathy (for specific symptoms)
- Oscillococcinum: take at first symptoms of a cold.
- Aconite: useful at onset of a cold when symptoms come on suddenly. Person is chilly, can have a fever, and has a fearful sensation of illness coming on.
- Allium cepa: cold with runny, clear nasal discharge.
- Pulsatilla: cold with yellow-green mucus, flushed, person may become more clingy and weepy.
- Hepar sulph: person has a stuffy sinus, chilly, and becomes very irritable.
- Nux vomica: person becomes chilly, constipated, and irritable.

Acupuncture/acupressure
- Press area between thumb and index finger where a mound of flesh pops out when these two fingers are pushed together laterally (LI-4) to relieve headache and head congestion. Also, push and hold LI-20 (this point located at the outside, lower corner of each nostril is to relieve sinus pressure.

Constitutional hydrotherapy
- Foot bath

Hepatitis

What it is: Different forms of hepatitis exist, but all are caused by viruses that infect the liver. (Please refer to Chapter 1 for more details.) In general, hepatitis A is spread through oral-fecal contamination. This commonly occurs as a result of a food preparer not washing his or her hands after going to the bathroom and then handling food. Hepatitis B is spread through sexual intercourse and infected blood products (including surgery, transfusion, and IV drug use). Hepatitis C is spread mainly through blood transfusions (rarer these days) and IV drug use. This type of hepatitis can lead to liver cirrhosis and liver cancer. Medical experts have also identified new forms of hepatitis, D, E and G, but are still gathering information on them.

Regardless of the type of hepatitis, these are common symptoms:

PHASE 1:
- *Malaise*
- *Fever*
- *Aversion to cigarettes*
- *Altered liver function tests*

PHASE 2:
- *Loss of appetite, nausea, vomiting*
- *Malaise*
- *Fever*
- *Weakness*
- *Headache*
- *Muscle ache*
- *Enlarged, tender liver*
- *Dark urine*
- *Occasionally, joint pain and hives*

PHASE 3: *(follows 3-10 days later)*
- *Dark urine and jaundice including the sclera (whites of the eyes); liver enlarged and mild spleen enlargement is present in 15-20 percent of patients*

A diagnosis of hepatitis is confirmed by blood tests, including antibody-antigen tests and elevated liver enzyme tests that signify liver inflammation.

TREATMENT PLANS FOR HEPATITIS

Herbal
- Milk thistle (85 percent silymarin): 150 mg, three times daily. Contains the active ingredient silymarin, which both protects liver cells from damage and promotes liver cell regeneration.
- Dandelion root: 30 drops or 500 mg, three times daily.
- Burdock root: 30 drops or 500 mg, three times daily.
- Phyllantharus amarus: 200 mg, three times daily
- Licorice root: 30 drops or 500 mg, three times daily.
- Reishi extract: 30 drops or 500 mg, three times daily.

Vitamins and Minerals
- Vitamin C: 3,000 mg daily minimum (aim for higher dosages that can be tolerated).
- *Intravenous* vitamin C by a doctor is highly advised.
- Selenium: 200 micrograms, twice daily.
- Multivitamin: daily.
- Vitamin B12 and folic acid injections by your doctor.
- B-complex: 50 mg to 100 mg daily.

Homeopathy (for specific symptoms)
- Chelidonium: useful to relieve jaundice.
- Natrum sulph: useful to relieve jaundice.
- Phosphorous: burning pain, high thirst for cold drinks, nausea, vomiting.
- Many others, depending on symptoms; see a practitioner trained in homeopathy.

Nutrition

- Plant-based diet.
- High-fiber diet, including foods healthy for the liver: dandelion greens, dandelion root, burdock root, mustard greens, black radish, apples, saffron, watercress, beets, parsley, artichokes, cherries, grapefruit, parsnips, endive, garlic, onion, chicory, carob, horseradish, kumquats, limes, quinces, grapes, wheat germ, lecithin, yogurt, tofu, soy, and ganoderma mushrooms.
- Fresh juicing: One apple, 1/4 beet, and three carrots is a good liver formula.
- Strict avoidance of alcohol, caffeine, tobacco, sugar products, saturated fats, meat, trans-fatty acids, hydrogenated oils (margarine, vegetable shortening, imitation butter spreads, most commercial peanut butters, oxidized fats), deep-fried foods, fast foods, and barbecue meats.

Other Treatment Plans

- Thymus extract—500 to 1,000 mg of thymus glandular daily or thymic protein A as prescribed by your physician.
- Constitutional hydrotherapy daily.
- Acupuncture/acupressure: Specific treatment by a practitioner can be very helpful in recovery from hepatitis and is highly recommended, along with Chinese herbal therapy.

HIV/AIDS

What it is: The conventional cause of AIDS is human immunodeficiency virus (HIV). HIV sabotages immunity so that the immune system (cell-mediated immunity) cannot protect itself from secondary infections. Unfortunately, a cure has yet to be found for AIDS. As discussed in Chapter 1, HIV interferes with T4 helper cells. These lymphocytes help other immune cells to increase in number to fight infections; T-4 inactivity leads to a suppression of the immune system. Blood is the most common medium of transmission (especially through sexual intercourse, IV needles, or being born to a mother who has HIV).

Common signs and symptoms include:

- *Persistent fever*
- *Weight loss*
- *Swollen lymph nodes*
- *Fatigue*
- *Dry cough*
- *Shortness of breath*
- *Night sweats*
- *Personality changes*
- *Diarrhea*

Opportunistic infections that threaten someone with AIDS include pneumocystis carinii pneumonia, candida albicans, toxoplasmosis, cryptosporidiosos, mycobacterium, and Kaposi's sarcoma (a type of cancer that is a later-stage complication and which has a poor prognosis).

The course and prognosis depends on the health of the infected person upon contracting the disease. Resulting infections are treatable, but unfortunately the course can be long and painful (physically and emotionally) for this incurable disease.

It is important to distinguish between AIDS and AIDS-related complex (ARC). Many ARC sufferers live relatively normal lives. Practicing a healthy lifestyle and dietary habits can often prevent ARC from progressing to AIDS. Some people with AIDS have managed to keep their condition at bay, while others have quickly declined.

Recent research demonstrates significant gains for patients using comprehensive alternative medical protocols as all or part of their treatment.

The diagnosis of HIV is made by a positive blood test for HIV antigens and antibodies. The diagnosis for AIDS depends on certain criteria:

- *Positive HIV test and a CD4 count (T helper cells) less than 200, or*
- *Percentage of T helper cells to total lymphocytes (CD8) less than 14 percent, or*
- *Presence of an opportunistic infection.*

Current conventional treatment focuses on the use of protease inhibitors and medications that interfere with the replication of the virus. Opportunistic infections are treated as they occur.

Natural therapies can be helpful to optimize immune function so that opportunistic infections or cancer, which are how people die from AIDS, do not occur.

TREATMENT PLANS FOR AIDS/HIV:

Herbal
- Licorice root *(Glycyrrhiza glabra):* small human studies have shown licorice root to be effective in maintaining healthy T helper and total T lymphocyte counts. It has also been used intravenously, with some success in reducing the viral load.[1-3] Dosage: 30 drops or 300 mg of an extract, three times daily.
- Reishi extract: 30 drops or 500 mg of an extract, three times daily.
- Maitake extract: 30 drops or 500 mg of an extract, three times daily.
- Chinese herbal therapy from a knowledgeable practitioner is strongly recommended.

145

Vitamins and Minerals
- Multivitamin: daily.
- Vitamin C: minimum of 1,000 mg, three times daily.
- Vitamin E (natural source): 400 to 800 IUs.
- Mixed carotenoid complex: 25,000 to 50,000 mg daily.
- Lipoic acid: 500 mg daily.
- Selenium: 200 micrograms daily.
- Vitamin B-12: 1 mg daily.
- B-complex: 50 mg, twice daily.
- IV-Vitamin C

Nutrition
- Diet should be a whole-foods diet high in vegetables, whole grains, legumes, nuts, and fresh fish and poultry. Avoid caffeine, alcohol, tobacco, sugar, fried foods, and trans-fatty acids such as margarine. Drink at least six 8-ounce glasses of purified water daily.

Homeopathy
- See a practitioner for individualized prescription.

Other Treatment Plans
- Thymus extract: 500 to 1,000 mg of thymus glandular daily, or thymic protein A as prescribed by your physician.
- Regular exercise.
- Stress reduction techniques such as prayer, tai chi, mental imagery, acupuncture.
- Constitutional hydrotherapy.

Herpes (type 1 and 2)

What it is: More than seventy viruses belong to the herpes family. The two most common types are herpes simplex (also known as HSV-1 or cold sores) and herpes complex (also known as HSV-2 or genital herpes). Genital herpes is spread through sexual contact. Herpes simplex is spread by direct skin contact with a person who has the virus (but may not have visible lesions). These reoccurring viral infections appear on the skin and mucous membranes (including lips, mouth, and genital area). A prodrome (warning) period occurs first, marked by tingling or itching, which is then followed by the eruption of clear fluid-filled vesicles. After a few days, the lesions dry up and form a crust. This can take two weeks or longer, depending on the individual. In both cases, the virus remains dormant until it is reactivated, usually by some sort of stress-inducer such as an infection, mental or physical pressure, or sun exposure. Genital herpes has a much higher reoccurrence rate than HSV-1, but both have similar natural treatments.

TREATMENTS FOR HERPES:

Herbal
- Lemon balm (*Melissa officinalis*) and licorice root (*Glycyrrhiza glabra*); both are available as topical creams and are helpful for many in reducing the severity of symptoms and duration of an outbreak for both types of herpes. Apply one or both of these twice daily to the lesions.

Vitamins and Minerals
- Vitamin C: 500 to 1,000 mg, four times daily.
- Bioflavonoids: 1,000 mg, three times daily.
- Selenium: 200 micrograms, twice daily with meals.
- Zinc: 50 mg daily.

Nutrition

- Avoid alcohol and refined sugar products. Also avoid foods that contain the amino acid arginine, because this amino acid may cause replication of HSV. Common foods containing arginine, include chocolate, peanuts, almonds, and other nuts. Do consume foods that contain lysine, an amino acid that helps suppress the herpes virus. Foods containing lysine include vegetables, legumes, turkey, potatoes, fish, and chicken.

Homeopathy (for specific symptoms)

- Herpes simplex nosode is useful for treating outbreaks and to prevent reoccurrences.
- Rhus toxicodendron: for pustular outbreaks that have a burning sensation.
- Natrum mur: good for chronic outbreaks and for people who break out when out in the sun.

Other Treatment Plans

- Applying ice to a cold sore at the first sign of symptoms works well to prevent an outbreak.
- Lysine: this amino acid is helpful for many people in preventing and treating herpes outbreaks. A typical adult dosage is 3,000 mg for the treatment and 1,500 mg for preventative purposes. It is best taken between meals.
- Thymus extract: 500 to 1,000 mg of thymus glandular daily, or thymic protein A as prescribed by your physician.

Measles

What it is: This viral condition (also known as rubeola or the nine-day measles) is a highly contagious infection that occurs during childhood. Common symptoms include fever, cough, malaise, runny nose, conjunctivitis (inflammation of the eye), and Koplik's spots (red spots with a bluish-white center that appear in the mouth). About three to five days after the onset of the symptoms, a rash typically appears. It begins on the neck and face and spreads to the trunk and then the rest of the body. A mild itch also develops.

Respiratory droplets spread the virus. Complications of measles can include pneumonia, ear infections, and other bacterial infections, and encephalitis (brain inflammation and swelling). The disease is usually self-limiting and runs its course in ten days. Conventional treatment includes the use of fever and pain relievers, and antibiotics when indicated.

TREATMENT PLANS FOR MEASLES

Note: Dosages are intended for children with a weight between twenty-five and forty pounds.

Herbal
- Echinacea: 15 to 30 drops, three times daily.
- Echinacea/goldenseal: 30 drops, three times daily, if a secondary bacterial infection is present.

Vitamins and Minerals
- Vitamin A: 100,000 IUs for three days and then 25,000 IUs for five days. Vitamin A use should be under the guidance of a doctor. A study of 180 children with rubeola (also known as nine-day measles) looked at vitamin A levels. Ninety-one percent of the children were found to have levels below normal. They were given vitamin A (200,000 IUs) supplements for two consecutive days. Results indicated an

149

eighty-seven percent decrease in death rate for children under two years of age.
- Vitamin C: 250 to 500 mg every three hours for immune system support and skin healing.

Nutrition
- Eat chicken soup, broths, and drink at least eight 8-oz glasses of water daily, eat also ginger, garlic, and onions for immune system support. Avoid sugary foods.

Homeopathy (for specific symptoms)
- Morbillinum-measles nosode: can help shorten the course and severity of the infection. Take as early as possible in the course of the infection.
- Pulsatilla: for a child who is often clingy, feverish, has low thirst, discharge from the eyes, and coughs at night.
- Sulphur: child is very warm, thirsty for cold drinks, and rash is red and itchy.

Other Treatment Plans
- Constitutional hydrotherapy

Mononucleosis (Epstein-Barr)

What it is: Mononucleosis is caused by the Epstein-Barr virus, a member of the herpes family of viruses. The virus replicates in the nasal and throat areas, then infects B-lymphocytes. Most adults have antibodies to Epstein-Barr virus. It is thought that this virus is harbored in the body during one's entire life. Only when the immune system is compromised does this virus replicate and cause disease. Signs of mono are fatigue, fever, sore throat, and swollen lymph nodes. The spleen enlarges in 50 percent of cases. The illness usually lasts an average of two weeks, but can last several weeks longer in some people. Transmission of the virus can occur through kissing, blood transfusion, or simply by drinking out of someone else's glass. Diagnosis is confirmed with blood work. Conventional treatment is typically a fever and pain reliever, like acetaminophen, and bed rest.

Note: Epstein-Barr is also associated with Burkitt's lymphoma. Cancer researchers feel that in susceptible persons, Epstein-Barr may initiate the development of Burkitt's lymphoma and other cancers. It is also believed to be an initiating factor for some people with chronic fatigue syndrome.

TREATMENT PLANS FOR MONONUCLEOSIS/EPSTEIN-BARR:

Herbal
- Echinacea-goldenseal combination: 20 to 30 drops or 500 mg every three hours.
- Olive leaf extract: 500 mg every three hours.
- Licorice root: 30 drops or 500 milligrams, three times daily. Acts as an antiviral.
- *Ceanothus americanus* (New Jersey tea): 30 drops or 500 mg, three times daily. Provides excellent help for an enlarged spleen.
- *Lomatium: 20–40 drops or 500 mg every three hours.*

NATURE'S VIRUS KILLERS

Vitamins and Minerals
- Vitamin C: 250 to 500 mg every three hours for immune system support and skin healing. Consider IU Vitamin C.
- Vitamin A: 25,000 IUs to 50,000 IUs daily.
- Vitamin B-complex: 50 mg daily.
- Zinc: 50 mg daily.

Nutrition
- Eat chicken soup, broths, and drink at least 8 oz of water daily. Eat ginger, garlic, and onions for immune-system support. Avoid sugary foods.

Homeopathy (for specific symptoms)
- Epstein-Barr virus homeopathic nosode: take at beginning of illness to reduce severity of symptoms and shorten duration.
- Gelsemium: muscle aches—feel as if bruised—extreme fatigue and dizziness.
- Arsenicum: intermittent fever, exhaustion, restlessness, chills, liver and spleen enlargement.
- Baptisia: muscle soreness, fever with chills.

Meningitis

What it is: Meningitis refers to an infection and inflammation of the membranes that cover the brain and spinal cord, known as the "meninges." It is usually caused by a viral or bacterial infection. Symptoms can include high fever, malaise, vomiting, dilated pupils, and a stiff neck and back. This can be a life-threatening infection and requires immediate hospitalization. The natural therapies included can be used as complementary approaches, especially for viral meningitis for which there are limited conventional treatments. Even though antibiotics are ineffective against viral infections, they are still prescribed for viral meningitis in case a bacterial infection is present. Antiviral drugs such as acyclovir are prescribed as well.

TREATMENT PLANS FOR MENINGITIS:

Herbal
- Oregon grape *(berberis)*: 60 drops or 500 mg of an extract, every two hours (use half-dose for children and a quarter for infants).
- Echinacea: 60 drops or 500 mg of an extract, every two hours (use half dose for children and a quarter for infants).
- Olive leaf: 60 drops or 500 mg of an extract, every two hours (use half dose for children and a quarter for infants).
- Astragalus: 60 drops or 500 mg of an extract, every two hours (use half dose for children and a quarter for infants).

Vitamins and Minerals
- Vitamin C: 1,000 mg every two hours, preferably by IV from your doctor.
- Vitamin A: 100,000 IUs for first two days and then 25,000 IUs until recovered.
- Zinc: 50 mg daily.

153

NATURE'S VIRUS KILLERS

Nutrition
- Eat chicken soup, broths, and drink 8 ounces of water daily. Eat ginger, garlic, and onions, foods that deliver immune-system support. Avoid sugary foods.

Homeopathy
- Belladonna: high fever, dilated pupils, flushed face. Best prescribed by a practitioner.

Other Treatment Plans
- Constitutional hydrotherapy.

Mumps

What it is: This childhood viral condition causes painful enlargement of the salivary glands, specifically the parotid glands which are located below the ears. The virus is spread through saliva and respiratory droplets. It usually occurs between the ages of five and fifteen. Symptoms usually include chills, headache, loss of appetite, and fever. After a day of these symptoms, parotid-gland swelling and pain occur. Complications are rare, although testicular swelling in boys can cause infertility if the disease occurs as a teenager or young adult. Conventional treatment calls for pain and fever relievers as well as bed rest.

TREATMENT PLANS FOR MUMPS:

Herbal
- Echinacea: 20 to 30 drops or 500 mg, every three hours.
- Olive leaf extract: 250 to 500 mg every three hours.

Vitamins and Minerals
- Vitamin C: 250 to 500 mg every three hours for immune system support.
- Vitamin A: 25,000 IUs daily.

Nutrition
- Eat chicken soup, broths, and drink at least 8 oz of water daily. Eat ginger, garlic, and onions for additional immune-system support. Avoid sugary foods.

Homeopathy (for specific symptoms)
- Belladonna: high fever, throbbing pain, flushed face.
- Pulsatilla: especially indicated for mumps that have spread to the testes.

Other Treatment Plans
- Constitutional hydrotherapy.
- Acupressure and acupuncture from a practitioner.

Pneumonia

What it is: This condition is caused by an infection of the lungs where the alveoli (tiny air sacs that line the lungs) become inflamed and filled with fluid. Various pathogens can infect the lungs, including viruses, bacteria, and mycoplasma. Symptoms of viral pneumonia include headache, fever, muscle pain, shortness of breath, and coughs that produce sputum. Pneumonia is often accompanied by an upper-respiratory infection. Antibiotics are ineffective against viral pneumonia. Bed rest and fluids are conventional recommendations. Diagnosis is made by listening to the lungs, through blood work, and by examining a chest X-ray.

Pneumonia is often preceded by an upper-respiratory infection. Although antibiotics are ineffective against viral diseases, they are often prescribed for viral pneumonia to treat or prevent a coexisting bacterial infection of the respiratory tract. Medical attention is necessary for pneumonia, whether it be viral or bacterial.

TREATMENT PLANS FOR PNEUMONIA:

Herbal
- Echinacea or echinacea-goldenseal combination: 60 drops or 500 mg, every three hours.
- Olive leaf extract: 500 mg, every three hours.
- Astragalus: 60 drops or 500 mg, every three hours.
- Mullein: 30 drops every three hours to soothe lung pain.

Vitamins and Minerals
- Vitamin C: 1,000 mg every three hours (cut back if diarrhea occurs) or IU Vitamin C.
- Vitamin A: 100,000 IUs daily for three days and then cut back to 50,000 IUs.
- Zinc: 50 mg daily.

Nutrition

- Eat chicken soup, broths, and drink at least 8 oz of water daily. Also eat ginger, garlic, and onions, which give immune-system support. Avoid sugary foods.

Homeopathy (for specific symptoms)

- Phosphorous: burning in lungs, feel better with cold drinks.
- Antimonium tart: lots of mucus in lungs, rattling of mucus in chest.
- Arsenicum: chills, restlessness, shortness of breath, fatigue.
- Sulphur: burning in lungs, hot and sweaty, last stage of pneumonia.
- Bryonia: sharp sticking pains in chest, chills.

Other Treatment Plans

- Acupuncture from a licensed practitioner.
- Chinese herbal therapy from a practitioner.
- Constitutional hydrotherapy.

Shingles

What it is: Known medically as herpes zoster, this condition is a reactivation of the varicella-zoster virus, the same virus that causes chicken pox. It lays dormant in the nerve endings and usually erupts after the age of fifty, generally when some event weakens the immune system. It usually begins with three or more days of chills, fever, and aches. By day four or five, crops of red, fluid-filled blisters appear on the skin. They usually occur on the abdomen and back, following the same contours as the ribs. They can occur anywhere on the body. Severe burning and itching can occur over the affected areas. This usually lasts two weeks, but the pain can go on for months. The lesions eventually scab over and resolve. Some people still have pain after the lesions are gone, a condition known as post-herpetic neuralgia.

Secondary infections can occur at the site of the blisters. Pain relievers and antiviral medications are the conventional treatment.

TREATMENTS FOR SHINGLES:

Vitamins and Minerals
- Vitamin C: 3,000 to 6,000 mg daily. For acute phases of the illness, IV vitamin C is recommended, given by a physician.
- Bioflavonoids: 3,000 mg daily.
- Selenium: 400 to 600 mg daily for acute treatment.
- Vitamin B-12 injections: 1cc daily or every two days by a physician.

Herbal
- Olive leaf extract: 500 mg four times daily.
- Echinacea: 60 drops or 500 mg, four times daily.
- Astragalus: 60 drops or 500 mg, four times daily.
- Lomatium: 30 to 60 drops or 500 mg, four times daily
- Capsaicin cream: extract of cayenne that inhibits pain. Apply topically to areas of pain.

159

Homeopathic (for specific symptoms)

- Variolinum: take at beginning of illness to shorten duration and severity.
- Arsenicum: burning pains made better with warm applications, restlessness.
- Rhus toxicodendron: burning pain, restlessness.
- Apis: burning and stinging pain. Made better with cold applications.

Other Treatment Plans

- Acupuncture.
- Chinese herbal therapy.
- Constitutional hydrotherapy.
- Thymus extract: 500 to 1,000 mg of thymus glandular daily, or thymic protein A as prescribed by your physician.

Sore Throat (Pharyngitis)

What it is: Throat infections are usually caused by viruses or bacteria. Fever, swollen lymph nodes, sore throat, and pain on swallowing are common symptoms. Conventional treatment is pain and fever relievers, and bed rest.

TREATMENT PLANS FOR SORE THROAT:

Herbal
- Echinacea: 60 drops or 500 mg, four times daily.
- Olive leaf extract: 500 mg, four times daily.
- Astragalus: 60 drops or 500 mg, four times daily.
- Lomatium: 30 to 60 drops or 500 mg, four times daily.
- Mullein, slippery elm, licorice root or marshmallow root to help soothe the throat: 30 to 60 drops or 500 mg, four times daily.

Vitamins and minerals
- Vitamin C: 1,000 mg every three hours (cut back if diarrhea occurs).
- Vitamin A: 100,000 IUs daily for three days, then cut back to 50,000 IUs.
- Zinc: 50 mg daily.

Nutrition
- Eat chicken soup, broths, and drink at least 8 ounces of water daily. Also eat ginger, garlic, and onions for added immune-system support. Avoid sugary foods.

Homeopathy (for specific symptoms)
- Phosphorous: raw burning pain in throat, feels better with cold drinks.
- Lycopodium: right-sided throat pain that feels better warm drinks.
- *Lachesis: left-sided sore throat with burning pain.*

161

Other Treatment Plans

- Acupuncture.
- Chinese herbal therapy.
- Throat hydrotherapy: alternate hot and cold compresses over throat area.
- Thymus extract: 500 to 1,000 mg of thymus glandular daily, or thymic protein A as prescribed by your physician.

Warts

What it is: Warts are caused by the human papilloma virus (HPV). Warts are commonly found on the hands, fingers, forearms, knees, and face. Warts on the soles of the feet and toes are known as plantar warts. Plantar warts are not known to spread to other areas of the body. Those on the genital area are called genital warts. They are highly contagious and transmitted sexually.

Caution: Certain strains of human papilloma virus that cause genital warts are associated with cervical cancer.

TREATMENT PLANS FOR WARTS:

Herbal
- Thuja oil: apply with a cotton swab to warts daily until they are gone.

Vitamins and Minerals
- Multivitamin: daily.
- Mixed carotenoids: 25,000 IUs daily.
- Selenium: 200 micrograms daily.
- Vitamin C: 1,000 mg three times daily.

Homeopathy
- Thuja: common homeopathic remedy used for warts.
- Indicated remedy is prescribed by practitioner.

Other Treatment Plans
- Acupuncture.
- Chinese herbal therapy.
- Thymus extract: 500 to 1,000 mg of thymus glandular daily, or thymic protein A as prescribed by your physician.
- Hypnosis and mental imagery have been shown to be effective in eliminating warts.

RECOMMENDED READING

Bennet, P and Barrie, S. 7-Day Detox Miracle. Rocklin, California: Prima Publishing, 1998.

Duke, J. *The Green Pharmacy.* Emmaus, Pennslyvania: Rodale Press, 1997.

Gazella, K. Activate Your Immune System. Green Bay, WI. Impakt Publications, 1999.

Murray, M. and Pizzorno, J. *Encyclopedia of Natural Medicine 2nd Ed.* Rocklin, California: Prima Publishing, 1998.

Stengler, Mark. *The Natural Physician: Your Guide for Common Ailments.* Burnaby, B.C., Canada: Alive Books, 1997.

Stengler, Mark. Echinacea: Supercharge Your Immune System. Green Bay, WI Impakt Publications, 1999.

Ullmal, R and Reicherg-Ulman, J. The Patient;s Guide to Homeopathic Medicine. Edmonds, WA. Picnic Point Press, 1995.

For more information on natural medicine, visit Dr. Stengler's WEbsite at www.thenaturalphysician.com.

Appendix I:
HYDROTHERAPY GUIDELINES

~~~~~~~~~~~~~~~~~~~~~~~~~~~~~~~~~~~~~~

Hydrotherapy is an effective technique that enhances the circulation of blood and lymph. It has been used successfully for two centuries.

As addressed in Chapter 9, the hot and cold techniques of hydrotherapy will trigger a fever reaction in the body and evoke an immune response. Fevers, as you may recall from earlier in this book, work in tandem with the immune system to eliminate viral infections.

Hydrotherapy also helps rid the body of toxins. Its ability to spur circulation helps the eliminatory organs (especially the liver and kidneys) excrete unwanted toxins.

This appendix describes two different hydrotherapy treatments that you can perform easily at home:

- *Constitutional hydrotherapy*
- *Foot hydrotherapy*

CONSTITUTIONAL HYDROTHERAPY

This form can be safely and easily done with or without assistance. Proper techniques accomplish these goals:

- *Detoxifying and purifying blood*
- *Enhancing circulation*
- *Optimizing digestion and the elimination processes*
- *Balancing the nervous system*
- *Assisting the immune system*

Step-by-step technique with assistance:

- Have the patient lie flat on his or her back.
- Soak a thick bath towel in hot water or heat it in a microwave. Wring out excess water and then place over the chest and abdomen areas. The temperature should be hot, but tolerable.
- Cover the patient's body with two large blankets to prevent chills. Allow the person to rest comfortably for five minutes.
- Remove the hot towel.
- Take a thin bath towel and soak it in cold water. Wring it out, but leave some moisture in the towel. Place this towel over the chest and abdomen areas. Place the blankets back over the body.
- Keep the cold towel on the area for ten to fifteen minutes.
- Have the person turn over and lie on his or her abdomen.
- Repeat the same hot and cold procedures.

Step-by-step technique without assistance:

- Take a hot shower or bath for 5 minutes.
- Step out of the stall or tub and dry quickly.
- Take the towel and run it under cold water. Wring it out and wrap it around you from your armpits to the groin area.
- Cover yourself with a wool blanket to prevent chilling.
- Keep the towel in place for twenty minutes, or until it is warmed.

Conditions helped by constitutional hydrotherapy:

Circulation problems: hemorrhoids, hypertension, Raynaud's disease, varicose veins

Digestion problems: constipation, Crohn's disease, diarrhea, heartburn, irritable bowel syndrome, peptic ulcer, ulcerative colitis

Female problems: infertility, menstrual cramping, PMS (pre-menstrual syndrome)

Male problems: impotence, prostate enlargement, prostatitis

Infections: bladder infections, colds, ear infections, the flu

Inflammatory problems: arthritis, lupus, multiple sclerosis, psoriasis

Respiratory problems: asthma, bronchitis, pneumonia, sore throat

FOOT HYDROTHERAPY

This treatment technique is best used for upper body congestion, because it draws blood flow toward the feet and lower extremities.

Step-by-step technique:

- Get a large bucket and fill it with water that is hot but tolerable.
- Soak both feet in this bucket for five to ten minutes.
- Lift your feet out of the bucket and dry them thoroughly.
- Soak a pair of white cotton socks in cold water and wring them out.
- Put on these wet socks.
- Cover the cotton socks with a pair of wool socks.
- Find a comfortable place to rest for about thirty minutes, and leave the socks on until they feel dry.

Recommended frequency for hydrotherapy techniques:

Acute conditions: one to two times a day.

Chronic conditions: three to five times a week, until condition is resolved.

Appendix II
HERBAL MEDICINE GUIDELINES

For newcomers to using herbs medicinally (and for others desiring a refresher course), information in this appendix will explain how to use botanicals safely and effectively.

Advantages of Herbal Medicines over Pharmaceutical Medications:

- *Herbs have fewer harmful side effects.*
- *Herbs cost less.*
- *Herbs treat both the symptoms and the underlying condition.*
- *Herbs help prevent illnesses.*
- *Herbs are versatile enough to be used for a variety of conditions.*

Herbal medicines come in many forms. Here are the major types:

Capsule. Dried herbs are placed inside a gelatinous capsule. Advantages: easy to take, standardized dosages that can be very potent.

Tea. Fresh or dried roots or leaves are brewed in hot water. The two brewing methods are *infusion* (usually one teaspoon of the herb's leaves are steeped in hot water for five to ten minutes); or *decoction* (usually one teaspoon of the herb's root boiled in water for ten to twenty minutes before ready to drink.) Advantages: good tasting, relaxing.

Tincture. Also known as extract, active compounds of an herb are converted into liquid form and preserved in an alcohol or glycerine solution. Advantages: easy to take.

Poultice. An herb is mixed with hot water or hot apple cider to form a paste. Dab olive oil on the affected skin area before applying this paste. (The poultice can also be sandwiched between two thin pieces of gauze and then onto the affected area.) Advantages: helps draw out irritants like bee venom and can be made if outdoors, using leaves of available medicinal herbs.

Compress. A clean cloth (made of cotton, wool, gauze, or linen) is soaked in a hot infusion or decoction of the liquid extract of the herb. This compress is then placed over the affected skin area and covered with plastic or wax paper to keep the compress warm. Advantages: helps draw out irritants in the affected area.

Liniment. Medicinal herbs are absorbed through the skin by means of massage. Advantage: works into the muscles quickly.

Essential oil. Medicinal herbs are pre-formulated to be highly concentrated by extracting the volatile oil portion. They can be applied topically or smelled for therapeutic effects. Advantages: goes to work on affected area.

Salve. Lanolin or oils are used as bases for topical application to form an insulating layer. Advantages: goes to work on affected area.

Cream. The desired herb is blended with an emulsion of water in oil. This allows this oily mixture to blend with skin secretions and penetrate the skin for healing purposes. Advantages: goes to work on affected area.

Decoding Product Labels

The explosion of new herbal products in health-food stores, pharmacies, and even your local supermarket can be daunting. So many choices. Which one is the right one for you? I recommend that you work closely with a naturopathic physician or a reputable herbalist who can help you pick the best herbs to meet your specific conditions. When shopping for these herbs at stores, here are some pointers:

- *Select products that list the full name of the herb. Ginseng, for instance, comes in three different types that treat different conditions.*
- *Make sure the label provides easy directions and recommended dosages.*
- *See if the manufacturer lists all ingredients in order of potency.*
- *Look to see if the specific parts of plants used are identified. Some herbs work better when their leaves are used; others house their medicinal ingredients in the roots, not the leaves.*
- *Buy only products that are wrapped in safety seals to prevent tampering and preserve freshness.*
- *Make sure the product lists an expiration date, lot number, toll-free hotlines, and Web addresses of manufacturers.*
- *Buy products that are certified organic to ensure no pesticides or herbicides were used in harvesting and preparing the plant for medicinal uses.*
- *Remember that reputable manufacturers list any cautions.*

Appendix III
SELECTING A HOLISTIC HEALTH PRACTITIONER

To contact the author:
Dr. Mark Stengler
9339 Genesee Ave., Suite 150,
LaJolla, CA
Phone: (619) 579-8681
Web site: www.thenaturalphysician.com

For a naturopathic doctor near you, contact:
American Association of Naturopathic Physicians
601 Valley Street, Suite 105
Seattle, WA 98109
Phone: (206) 298-0126
Fax: (206) 298-0129
Web site: www.naturopathic.org

For homeopathy, contact:
National Center for Homeopathy
801 North Fairfax Street, Suite 306
Alexandria, VA 22314
www.healthy.net/nch

For acupuncture, contact:
American Association of Oriental Medicine
433 Front Street
Catasauqua, PA 18032
Phone: (610) 266-1433
(888) 500-7999 (toll-free)
www.aaom.org

NOTES

~~~~~~

CHAPTER 1

1. Bellanti M.D., Joseph A., *Immunology III*, 2nd Ed., Philadelphia: W. B. Saunders Company, 1985.
2. Claude Bennet M.D., J.; Smith Jr. M.D., Lloyd H.; and Wyngaarden M.D., James B., *Cecil Textbook of Medicine*, 19th Ed., Philadelphia: W. B. Saunders Company, 1992, pp. 1798–1806.
3. Cotran M.D., Ramzi S.; Kumar M.D., Vinay; Robbins M.D., Stanley L.; Schoen M.D. Ph.D., Frederick J., *Robbins: Pathologic Basis of Disease*, 5th Ed., Philadelphia: W. B. Saunders Company, 1994, pp. 315–319.
4. Claude Bennet M.D., J. Smith Jr. M.D., Lloyd H. and Wyngaarden M.D., James B., Cecil Textbooks of Medicine, 19th Ed. Philadelphia: W.B. Sanders Company, 1992, pg. 1801–1804.

CHAPTER 2

1. Fishbach F., *A Manual of Laboratory and Diagnostic Tests*, 4th Ed., Philadelphia: J. B. Lippincott Company, 1992, pp. 25–39.
2. Schauf, C. et al. *Human Physiology*. St. Louis, Missouri: Times Mirror/Mosby College Publishing, 1990.
3. Claude Bennet M.D., J. Smith Jr. M.D., Lloyd H.; and Wyngaarden M.D., James B., *Cecil Textbook of Medicine*, 19th Ed., Philadelphia: W. B. Saunders Company, 1992, p. 1799.

1. Farnsworth N. et al., "Medicinal plants in therapy," Bull World Health Org., 63, 1985, pp. 965–981.
2. Stengler, M., *The Natural Physician*. Burnaby, Canada: Alive Books, 1997, p. 154.
3. Murray, M. T. *Better Nutrition*. December 1998 p. 12.
4. *Whole Foods Natural Herbal Sales Survey,* October 1998 pp. 19–20.
5. Hobbs, Christopher., *Echinacea: The Immune Herb,* Santa Cruz: Botanica Press. 1990, p.12.
6. Bauer, R., and Wagner, H., "Echinacea species as potential immunostimulatory drugs," *Econ Med Plant Res 5.* 1991 pp. 288–289.
7. Schoenberger, D., "The influence of immune stimulating effects of a pressed juice from Echinacea purpurea on the course and severity of colds," results of a double-blind study, *Forum Immunologie* 8, 1992 pp. 2–12.
8. Hoheisel, O.; Sandberg, M.; Bertram, S., et al., "Echinagard treatment shortens the course of the common cold: a double blind placebo controlled clinical trial." *Eur J Clin Res* 9. 1997 pp. 261–268.
9. Brauning, B. et al., "Echinacea purpurea radix for strengthening the immune response in flu like infections," *Zeit Phytother* 12, 1992, pp. 7-13.
10. Jurcic, K. et al., "Two test subject studies for the stimulation of granulocyte phagocytosis by echinacea-containing preparations." *Zeit Phytother* 10(2), 1989 pp. 67–70, .
11. Berg, A. et al. "Influence of Echinacin (EC31) treatment on the exercise-induced immune response in athletes," *J. Clin Res* 1, 1998, pp. 367–380.
12. Ondrizek, R. R. et al., "Inhibition of human sperm mortility by specific herbs used in alternative medicine." *J Assist Reprod. Genet* 16. Feb. 1999, pp. 87–91.
13. Bensky, D., and Gamble, A., *Chinese Herbal Medicine: Materia Medica,* Rev. Ed. Seattle: Eastland Press, 1993.pp. 319–320.
14. Huang, Z.Q.; Qin, N. P.; Ye, W., "Effect of Astragalus membranaceus on T-lymphocyte subsets among patients with

viral myocarditis." *Chung Kuo Chung HSI I Chich Ho Tsa Chih* 15. 1995, pp. 328–330.

15. Zhao, K.W., and Kong H.Y., "Effect of Astragalan on secretion of tumor necrosis factor in human peripheral mononuclear cells," *Chung Kuo Chung HSI I Chich Ho Tsa Chih* 13. pp. 263–265, 1993.

16. Wang, Y.; Qian X. J.; Hadley, H. R.; Lau, B. H., "Phytochemicals potentiate interleukin 2 generated lymphokine activated killer cell cytotoxicity against morine renal cell carcinoma," *Mol Biother* 4, 1992, pp. 143–46.

17. Chu, D. T.; Lin, J. R.; Wong W. "The in vitro potentiation of LAK cell cytotoxicty in cancer and AIDS patients induced by F-3-a fractionated extract of Astragalus membranaceus." *Chung Hua Chung Liu Tsa Chih* 16, 1994 pp. 167–171.

18. Chang, H. M., and P. Hui-Hay But, *Pharmacology and Applications of Chinese Materia Medica,* Vol. 1, Singapore: World Scientific, 1986.

19. Hobbs, C. Medicinal Mushrooms. Loveland, Colorado: Botanica Press, 1998, pp. 96–107.

20. Walker, Morton, "Antimicrobial Attributes of Olive Leaf Extract," *Townsend Letter for Doctors and Patients,* July 1996, No. 156, pp. 80–85.

21. Abe, N. Ebina, T.; and Ishida, N., "Interferon induction by glycyrrhizin and glycyrrhetinic acid in mice," *Microbial Immunol* 26, 1982, pp. 535–539.

22. Pompei, R. et al., "Antiviral activity of glycyrrhizic acid." *Experentia* 36. 1980, pp. 304–305.

23. Zakay-Rones et al., "Inhibition of several strains of influenza virus in vitro and reduction of symptoms by an elderberry extract (Sambucus nigra L.) during an outbreak of influenza B in Panama," *Journal of Alternative and Complementary Medicine,* 1(4), 1995 pp. 361–369.

24. Gallo, M. et al., "Pregnancy Outcome Following Gestational esposure to Echinacea, A Prospective Controlled Stud." The Motherisk Program, Division of Clinical Pharmacology, Hospital for Sick Children and the University of Toronto, and the Canadian College of Naturopathic Medicine, 1999.

CHAPTER 4

1. Quillin, P., *Beating Cancer with Nutrition,* Tulsa: The Nutrition Times Press, Inc., 1994, p. 37.
2. U.S. Environmental Protection Agency, *1987–1994 Toxic Release Inventory National Report,* Washington, D. C.: Office of Toxic Substances.
3. Passwater, R., *Trace Elements, Hair Analysis, and Nutrition.* New Canaan, Connecticut.: Keats Publishing, 1983.
4. White, D. M., et al., "Neurologic syndrome in 25 workers from an aluminum smelting plant." *Arch Int Med* 152. 1992, pp. 1443–1448.
5. Holtzman, R. B., and Flcewicz, F. H. "Lead-210 and polmium-210 in tissues of cigarette smokers," *Science* 153, 1996, pp. 1259–1260.
6. Siblerud, R. L., "The relationship between mercury from dental amalgam and mental health," *American Journal of Psychotherapy,* October 18, 1989, pp. 575–587.
7. Hikino H., Kiso Y.; Wagner, H.; and Fiebig. "Antihepatotoxic actions of flavolignans from Silybum marianum fruits." *Planta Medica* 50, 1984 pp. 248–250.

CHAPTER 5

1. Patterson B. H., Block, G. *American Journal of Public Health* 78. March 1988, p. 282.
2. Bloch, A., Thomson, C. "Position of The American Dietetic Association: phytochemicals and functional foods." *Journal of American Dietetic Assocation.* 95, 1995, p. 93–496.
3. Weber, N. D., et al., "In vitro virucidal effects of Allium sativum (garlic) extract and compounds." *Planta Medica* 58, 1992, pp. 417–423.
4. Simopoulos, A., *The Omega Plan,* New York: HarperCollins, 1998, p. 5.
5. Thompson, L. U., et al., "Mammalian lignan production from various foods." *Nutr Cancer* 16. 1991, pp. 43–52.
6. Setchell, K. D. R., and Adlercreutz, H., "Mammalian lignans and phytoestrogens: Recent studies on their formation,

metabolism, and biological role in health and disease." *Role of Gut Flora in Toxicology and Cancer,* Rowland, I.R. Ed. London: Academic Press, 1988, pp. 315–43.

7. Sanchex, A.; Reeser, J.; Lau, H., et al. "Role of sugars in human neutrophilic phagocytosis." *American Journal of Clinical Nutrtion* 26, 1973, pp. 1180–1184.

8. Ringsdorf, W., Cheraskin, E., and Ramsay R., "Sucrose, neutrophilic phagocytosis and resistance to disease." *Dent Surv* 52, 1976 pp. 46–48.

9. Bernstein, J; Alpert S.; Nauss, K.; and Suskind R. "Depression of lymphocyte transformation following glucose ingestion." *American Journal of Clinical Nutrition* 30, 1977 pp. 613.

10. Smith, B. "Organic foods versus supermarket foods: Element levels," *J Appl Nutr* 45, 1993, pp. 35-39.

11. Newberne, P., and Conner, M. W., "Food Additives and Contaminants: An update," *Cancer* 58, 1986, pp. 1851–1862.

CHAPTER 6

1. Hasselbacj, H. et al., "Decreased thymus size in formula fed infants compared to breast-fed infants," *Acta Periactr* 85, 1996 pp. 1029–1032.

2. Beardsley, T.; Pierschbacher, M.; Wetzel, G. D.; Hays, E. F. "Induction of T-cell maturation by a cloned line of thymic epithelium (TEPI)," *Proc Natl Acad Sci* 80, 1983, p. 6005.

3. Cazzola, P.; Mazzanti, P.; and Bossi, G., "In vivo modulating effect of a calf thymus acid lysate on human T lymphocyte subsets and CD4/CD* ratio in the course of different diseases." *Current Therapeutic Research* 42, 1987 pp. 1011–1017.

4. Koutabb, N. M.; Prada, M.; and Cazzola P. "Thymodulin: Biological properties and clinical applications." *Medical Oncology and Tumor Pharacotheropy* 6, 1989 pp. 5–9.

5. Galli, M. et al., "Attempt to treat acute type B Hepatitis with an orally administered thymic extract (Thymomodulin): Preliminary results. *Drug Experimental Clinical Research* 11, 1985, pp. 665–669.

6. Bortolotti, F., et al. "Effect of an orally administered thymic derivative, Thymodulin, in chronic type B hepatitis in children." *Current Therapeutic Research* 43, 1988, pp. 67–72.
7. Valesini, G. et al., "A calf thymus lysate improves clinical symptoms and T cell defects in the early stages of HIV infection: Second report," *Eur. J Cancer Clin Oncol* 23, 1987 pp. 1915–1919.
8. Mulder, J. W., et al., "Dehydroepiandosterone as predictor for progression to AIDS in asymptomatic human immunodeficiency virus type infected men," *Journal of Infectious Diseases* 165, 1992, pp. 413–418.
9. Gordon, G. B., et al., "Serum levels of dehydroepiandrosternoe and its sulfate and the risk of developing bladder cancer," *Cancer Res* 51, 1991 pp. 1366–69.
10. Irwin, M.; Mascovich, A.; Gillin J. C., et al., "Partial sleep deprivation reduces natural killer cell activity in humans," *Psychom Med* 56(6). pp. 493–498.

CHAPTER 7

1. Patterson, B. H., and Block, G., *American Journal of Public Health* 78, March 1988, p. 282.
2. *Pennington, J., and Schoen, S., "Total Diet Atudy: Estimated Dietary INtakes of Nutritional Elements, 1982–1991. Int. J Vitamin Nutr. Res. 66,(4) 1996, pp. 350–362.*
3. Sembda, R. D. Vitamin A, immunity, and infection. *Clin Inf Dis* 19. 1994, pp. 489–499.
4. *JAMA* 269. pp. 898-903, 1993.
5. Fawzi, W. W. et al., Vitamin A Supplementation and Child Mortality. A Meta-Analysis. JAMA 269, 1943, pp. 898-903.
6. Arrieta, A.C., et al. "Vitamin A levels in children with measles in Long Beach, Ca. J pediatr" 121. pp. 75-78, 1992.
7. Semba, R.D., et al. "Increased mortality associated with vitamin A deficiency during human immunodeficiency virus type 1 infection." *Arch Intern Med* 153. pp. 2149-2154, 1993.
8. Beisel, W.; Edelman, R.; Nauss, K.; and Suskind, R., "Single nutrient effects of immunologic functions." *JAMA* 245, 1981, pp. 53–58.

9. Palteil, P. O. et al., "Clinical correlates of subnormal vitamin B12 levels in patients infected with the human immunodeficiency virus," *American Journal of Hematology* 49, 1995 pp. 318–322.

10. Weinberg, J. B., et al., "Inhibition of productive human immunodeficiency virus-1 infection by cobalamins," *Blood* 86, 1995, pp. 1281–1287.

11. Bendich, A. "Vitamin C and immune responses," *Food Technol* 41, 1987 pp. 112–114.

12. Frei, B.; England, L.; and Ames, B. N. "Ascorbate is an outstanding antioxidant in human blood plasma," *Proc Natl Acad Sci* 86, 1989, pp. 6377–6381.

13. Ginter, E. "Optimum intake of vitamin C for the human organism," *Nutr Health* 1, 1982, pp. 66–77.

14. Cathart, R.F. "The third face of vitamin C," *J Orthomol Med* 7, 1992, pp. 197-200.

15. *J Orthomol Psychiat* 10, 1981 p.p 125–132.

16. Klenner, F. R. "Observations on the dose of administration of ascorbic acid when employed beyond the range of a vitamin in human pathology," *J Applied Nutr* 23, 1971, pp. 61–68.

17. Baur, H., and Staub, H. "Treatment of hepatitis with infusions of ascorbic acid: Comparison with other therapies," *JAMA* 156, 1985, p. 565.

18. Murray, Michael. *Encyclopedia of Nutritional Supplements.* Rocklin, California: Prima Publishing. p.p. 44–45, 1996.

19. Kiremidjiian-Schumacher, L. et al. "Supplementation with selenium and human immune cell functions; II. Effect on cytotoxic lymphocytes and natural killer cells," *Biol Trace Elem Res* 41, 1994, pp. 115–127.

20. Dardenne, M., et al., "Contribution of zinc and other metals to the biological activity of the serum thymic factor," *Proceedings of the National Academy of Sciences,* 79, 1982, pp. 5370–5373.

21. Folkers, K. et al., "Increase in levels of IgG in serum of patients treated with coenzyme Q10," *Research Communications in Chemical Pathology Pharmacology,* 1982.

22. Stengler, M., *The Natural Physician, Burnaby, Canada: Alive Books, 1997.*

CHAPTER 8

1. Stengler, M., *The Natural Physician*, Burnaby, Canada: Alive Books, 1997.
2. Morrison, R., *Desktop Guide to Keynotes and Confirmatory Symptoms*, Albany, New York: Hahnemann Clinic Publishing, 1993.

CHAPTER 9

1. Lipton, Douglas: Lincoln Clinic Study; Konefal, Janet: Miami Study; Bullock, Milton: Hennepin County Study. U.S. Dept. of Health and Human Services, National Institutes of Health; Office of Human Services, AM, Vol. 1, No. 3, January 1994.
2. Brewington, Vincent et al., "Acupuncture as a Detoxification Treatment: An Analysis of Controlled Research," *Journal of Substance Abuse Treatment*, Vol. 11, No. 4, 1994, pp. 289–307.
3. "Jayasuriya: Paper for the 5th World Congress of Acupuncture," Tokyo: Japan, 1977.

CHAPTER 10

1. Ikegami, N., et al. "Prophylactic Effects of Long Term Oral Administration of Glycyrrhizin on AIDS Development of Asymptomatic Patients." International Conference on AIDS 9(1) 1993:234 (abstract no. PO-A25-0596).
2. Ikegami, N. et al. "Clinical Evaluation of Glycyrrhizin on HIV infected Asymptomatic Hemophiliac Patients in Japan." Fifth International Conference on AIDS (June 1989): Abstract W.B.P. 298; cited in *AIDS Treatment News* 103 (May 18, 1990), 54.
3. Mori, K., et al. "Effects of Glycyrrhizin (SNMC: Strogner Neominophagen C) in Hemophilia Patients with HIV-1 Infection." Tohoku Journal Experimental Medicine 162. pp. 183-193, 1990.

GLOSSARY OF TERMS

Absorption. The passage of nutrients from the digestive system into the bloodstream.

Acupressure. This natural therapy uses finger and hand pressure on specific points on the body to relieve pain, reduce symptoms of illness, and promote health.

Acupuncture. This component of Chinese medicine involves the insertion of needles into specific points in the body for therapeutic reasons. It may also involve the use of pressure, heat, or electromagnetic energy to stimulate anatomic acupuncture points in the body. It is based on the theory that the body has several main energy channels that can be blocked or interrupted by illness or disharmony.

Adaptogen. A substance that helps the body to increase its resistance to mental or physical stress. It also has a balancing effect on body processes.

Adrenal glands. A pair of glands located at the top of the kidneys. These glands produce stress hormones such as epinephrine, cortisol, and DHEA, among others.

Allicin. A biologically active ingredient found in garlic.

Alpha-linolenic acid. An essential fatty acid of the omega-3 group, found in fish, fish oils, and certain plants such as flax seed.

Amino acids. Consist of twenty individual building blocks of protein. Each amino acid can produce different biochemical effects.

Antibodies. Large proteins of the blood and body fluids that are produced by the immune system in response to foreign invaders.

Antigen. Any parts of bacteria, toxins, or foreign proteins that enter the body and provide an immune response that results in the formation of antibodies.

Anti-inflammatory. Any substance that lessens or blocks swelling.

Antioxidant. Any substance that protects other cells from oxidation or free-radical damage. The best known antioxidants include vitamins A, C, and E, beta-carotene, and selenium.

Astringent. Any substance that binds or constricts.

ATP (adenosine triphosphate). The energy currency of cells.

Autoimmune condition. This occurs when the body's immune system reacts against its own tissues and inflicts damage on them.

Bioflavonoids. A vitamin-like supplement that displays abilities similar to vitamin C. They are obtained from the pigments of flowers and fruits, such as orange and lemon peels.

B-lymphocytes. A special group of white blood cells that manufactures specific antibodies to pathogens with which they come in contact.

Carbohydrates. Starchy and sugary foods.

Carcinogens. Cancer-causing substances.

Carotenoids. A group of 600-plus naturally occurring pigments found in nature in certain fruits and vegetables, which function as antioxidants and precursors for vitamin A.

Catecholamines. The hormones in the adrenal glands that have a fight-or-flight response.

Chelating agent. A chemical that binds to something. For example, EDTA is used in chelation therapy to bind and pull out heavy metals, like lead.

Cholesterol. A fat-soluble substance necessary for proper cell functions. Excessive amounts of cholesterol can be harmful.

Collagen. Protein that is the main ingredient of connective tissue.

Creatine. A nutrient that occurs naturally within the body. It is composed of three amino acids—arginine, glycine, and methionine.

Corticosteroids. Hormones released by the adrenal glands during times of stress.

Cortisol: A stress-response hormone produced by the adrenal glands.

DHEA (dehydroepiandosterone): A hormone produced by the adrenal glands that serves as the precursor to many of the hormones within the body. This hormone is being studied for its effect on chronic illnesses (such as arthritis and lupus) and hormone-deficiency illness.

DNA (deoxyribonucleic acid). A substance contained in cells. It provides the genetic code.

Diuretic. A substance that increases the excretion of urine.

Enzyme. A catalyst for biochemical reactions in the body and an aide for digestion.

NATURE'S VIRUS KILLERS

Essential fatty acids. Substances required for normal bodily function, which the body cannot produce on its own. They include linoleic and linolenic acid.

Fat-soluble. Cannot be dissolved in water, only in fats and oils. Fat-soluble vitamins are A, D, K, and E. All need fat to be properly absorbed.

Flavonoids. A group of antioxidant plant pigments that provides the colors for fruits and flowers.

Food allergy. A reaction to a food that invokes an immune response. Symptoms can include hives, anaphylaxis (closing of the windpipe), runny nose, and stomach problems.

Food sensitivity. A reaction to a food that does not cause a considerable immune-system reaction. Common symptoms are rashes, digestive problems, headaches, mood swings, and insomnia.

Free radical. A highly reactive molecule with an unpaired electron that can damage cells and tissues. Formed from heated oils and fats, environmental pollution, and as a by-product of metabolic reactions within the body. Free radicals are neutralized by antioxidants and naturally occurring enzymes in the body.

Glutamine. An amino acid.

Glutathione. A protein composed of the amino acids cysteine, glutamic acid, and glycine. It possesses antioxidant properties and helps the liver in detoxification.

Gluten. The primary protein found in certain grains, including barley, oats, rye, and wheat.

Glycine. An amino acid that is used in detoxification.

188

Goldenseal (*Hydrastis canadensis*). An herb that possesses immune-system enhancing properties and antibacterial properties.

Grape seed extract. A substance that contains PCOs (procyanidolic oligomers), a group of plant flavonoids known to provide many health benefits. PCOs exert potent effects to protect body cells and tissues from oxidative damage. Grape seed extract works against allergies, and cardiovascular disease by enhancing the immune and circulatory systems.

Herbal medicine. The use of different parts of plants (usually leaves, roots, flowers, and rhizomes) to treat symptoms and promote health. The medicinal use of herbs dates back centuries.

Histamine. A special chemical secreted by cells to alert the immune system.

Homeopathy. A natural medicine treatment involving remedies made from plant, animal, or mineral substances that are highly diluted. The aim is to stimulate the body just enough to trigger a healing response. It is based on the principle that "like cures like."

Hydrogenation. The process used to make margarine out of vegetable oils by transforming certain fatty acids.

Hydrotherapy. This technique involves the use of hot and cold water applications in various ways to ease a variety of health conditions.

Imagery and visualization: This natural therapy relies upon the use of thoughts to deal with pain, control illness, and attain goals.

Immune system: The body's defense system, which protects against viruses and other foreign substances and organisms.

Immunoglobulins. Antibodies produced by B-lymphocytes in response to foreign proteins or antigens.

Indole-3-carbinol. A chemical compound found in certain vegetables that activates detoxifying enzymes.

Inflammation. The body's reaction to tissue injury. Typical reactions include redness, swelling, heat, and pain.

Interferon. A special chemical secreted by cells when they become infected with viruses. Interferon alerts natural killer cells to step up their activity. Also helps other cells to better resist viral attacks.

IU. International unit, a type of measurement for certain vitamins.

Isoflavone. A type of flavonoid.

Lactose. A type of sugar (disaccharide) found in cows' milk.

Leaky gut. A condition that occurs when damage to the intestinal barrier allows normal and toxic bowel components to leak into the body.

Lecithin. A phospholipid mixture of fatty acids, glycerol, phosphorus, choline, and inositol that is a normal part of the cell membrane.

Lentinan. An active ingredient in shiitake mushrooms that stimulates the immune system, suppresses viral carcinogens, attacks cancers, and prevents cancer from recurring after surgery.

Licorice root. An antiviral herb that supports the immune system and inhibits many viruses.

Linoleic acid. An essential fatty acid that provides some anti-inflammatory properties for the body. Found in black currant, borage, corn oils, evening primrose, safflower, and sunflower.

190

L-Tryptophan. An essential amino acid that is necessary for proper development and growth. It serves as the precursor to the brain chemical serotonin, which is involved in mood enhancement.

Lymphatic system. A complex network of thin, vein-like tubes that run parallel to blood vessels in the body. This system performs numerous functions, including the draining of wastes from tissues and the filtering out of debris and toxins.

Lymphocyte. A group of white blood cells that includes the B cells, the T cells, and natural killer cells.

Lysine. An amino acid necessary for growth. It has an inhibitory effect on the herpes simplex virus.

Macrophages. Cells within the body that act like garbage collectors whenever they encounter pathogenic agents.

Malabsorption. Defective absorption of nutrients by the intestines into the bloodstream. Improper absorption of foods can lead to a buildup of disease-producing toxins in the body.

Metabolism. The chemical changes in living cells by which energy is produced for vital processes and activities.

Methionine. An amino acid necessary for detoxification and growth.

Mineral. An inorganic element or compound that occurs naturally. The body cannot synthesize its own minerals, but they are needed for the proper function of vitamins and other enzyme systems.

Monounsaturated fat. A fatty acid that lacks two hydrogen atoms and has one double bond between carbons. Olive oil is an example.

Mucus membranes. The inside lining of body cavities, such as the respiratory and digestive tracts.

N-Acetylcysteine. An amino acid complex that is used to detoxify heavy metals and dissolve mucus from the body.

Naturopathic doctor. A physician trained in conventional and natural medicine at a four-year medical school. These professionals focus on treatments that emphasize the body's inherent healing mechanisms.

Natural killer cells. A type of white blood cells that attacks pathogens. They are the body's first line of attack against cancerous cells.

Neurotransmitter. A chemical nerve impulse used by the brain and the nervous system for communication.

Nosode. A homeopathic remedy made from a diseased tissue or the disease itself to prevent or treat the associated disease. For example, herpes virus made into a homeopathic nosode can be used to prevent or treat a case of herpes. Similar in concept to that of a vaccine, but in this case using homeopathic preparations.

Nutrient. A substance required by the body for growth and to maintain life.

Organic. Refers to any foods grown without pesticides, herbicides, hormones, or other chemicals.

Oxidation. The process in which a substance either combines with oxygen or loses an electron.

Pathogen. A disease-producing microorganism.

Pectin. A fiber found in fruits (also available in supplements) that increases the secretion of digestive enzymes.

Phagocytes. A group of immune cells that surrounds and destroys unwanted cells and substances.

Phospholipids. A type of fat found in cell membranes that provides protection from chronic exposure to organic solvents (especially in the liver).

Phytoestrogens. Plant estrogens, chemicals found in some foods and herbs.

Plant enzymes. Purified enzymes obtained from plant sources that are commonly used as digestive aides.

Prostaglandins. Hormone-like molecules that help control inflammation in the body.

Proteases. Protein-splitting enzymes.

Protein. A combination of amino acids necessary to the body for forming tissues, enzymes, and hormones, and for the creation of energy.

Quercitin. A bioflavonoid used as a natural antihistamine.

Rhizome. Plant roots that extend underneath or above the ground.

Rutin. A flavonoid that acts as a scavenger for unwanted viral invaders and provides the body with defense against colds and upper respiratory infections.

Saturated fat. A type of fat with the maximum number of bonded hydrogens. It is solid at room temperature and is found in animal and dairy products. Associated with increased risk of cancer, heart disease, and inflammatory diseases.

Serotonin. A neurotransmitter made from tryptophan.

T cells. A group of lymphocytes that originates in the thymus and helps with cell-mediated immunity.

Thymus. The principal gland of the immune system, located behind the breastbone.

Toxin. A poison arising from internal production (malabsorption in the digestive tract) or from the environment (air, water, food).

Triglyceride. A compound that consists of three fatty acids and glycerol. It can be a fat in the blood or diet.

Tyrosine. An amino acid that is a precursor to neurotransmitters. It is used for depression and hypothyroidism conditions.

Unsaturated fats. A fat that is liquid at room temperature and is a primary component of essential fatty acids such as flaxseed oil.

Vitamin. An organic substance required for body function. People can synthesize some vitamins, but the rest must be obtained through the diet or supplementation.

Water-soluble. The ability to dissolve in water. For instance, vitamin C is water-soluble and does not need fat to be absorbed in the body.

INDEX